My Personal M

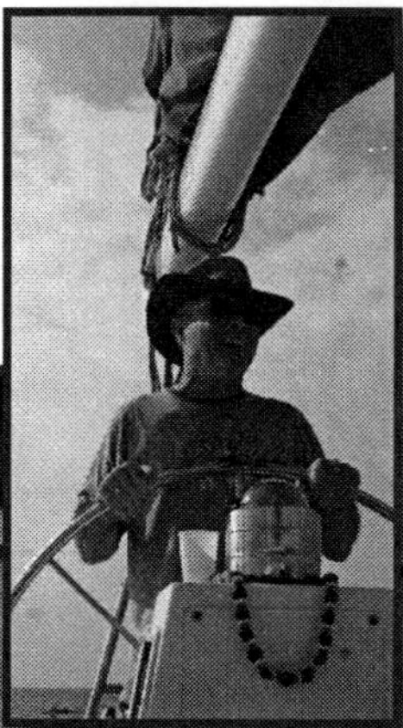

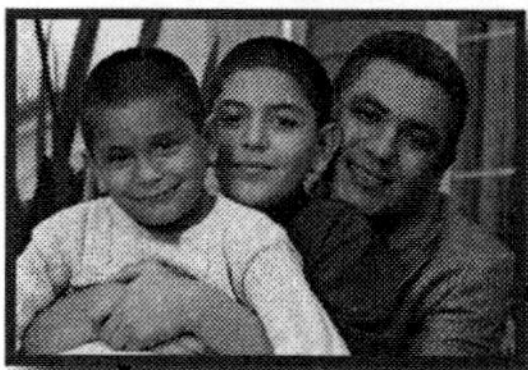

Personal Health Managemen

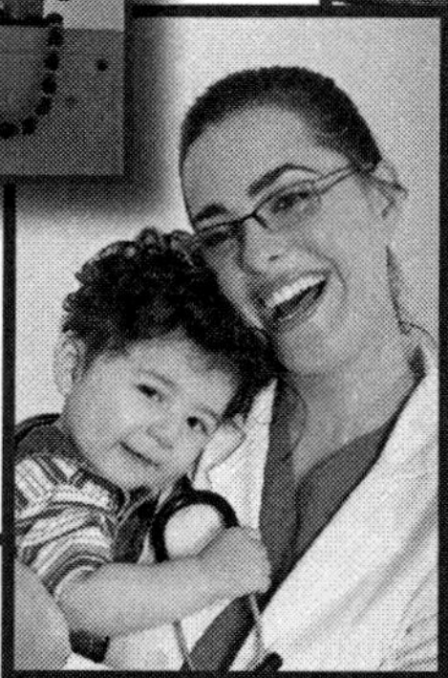

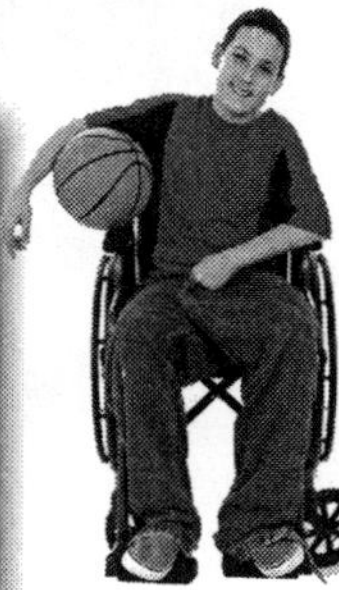

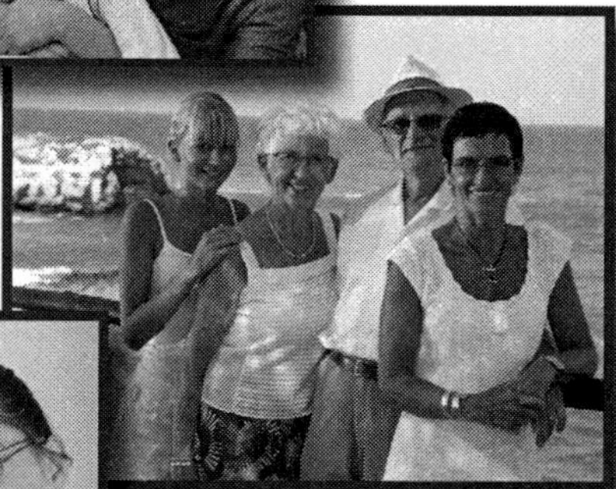

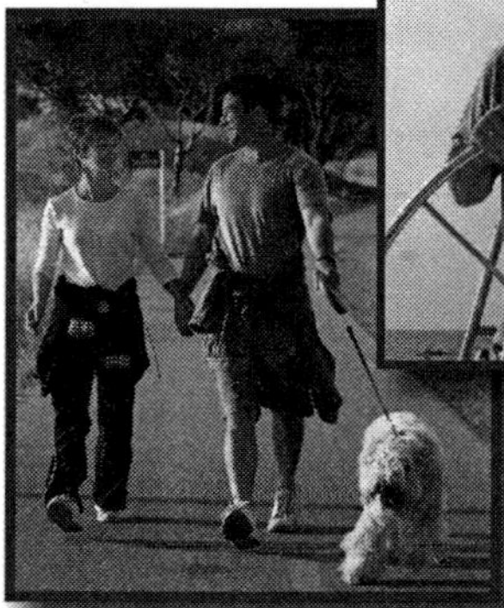

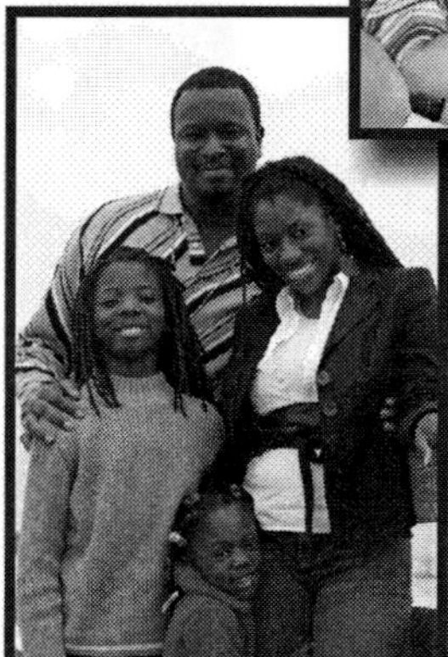

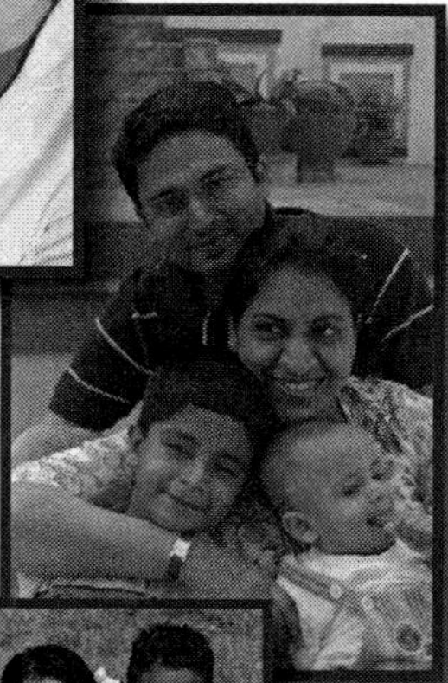

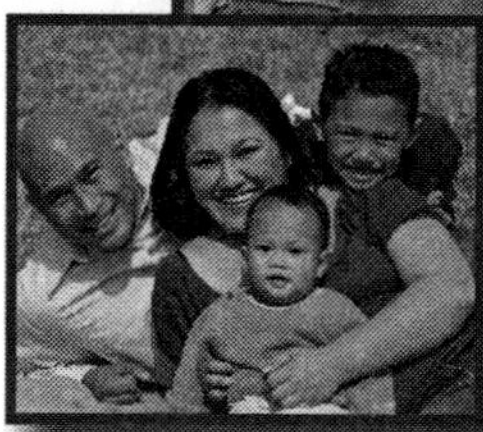

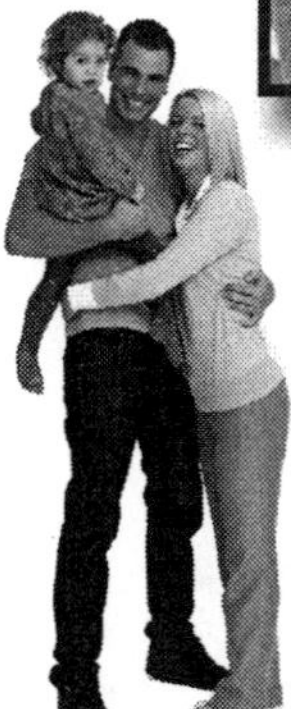

Recommended by Physicians, Dentists and Service Providers

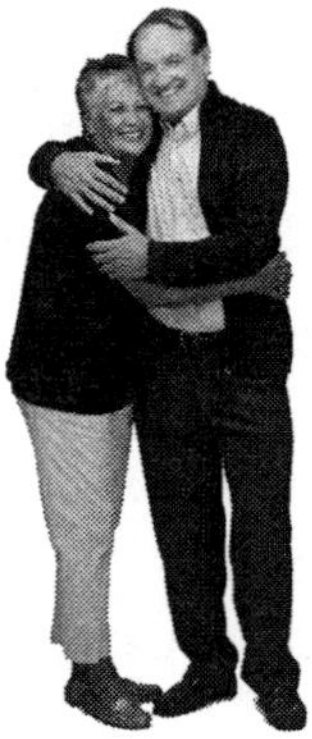

NAME

My Personal Medical Journal

If I have misplaced this journal, please contact me or forward it to:

Name ______________________________

Address ______________________________

Phone (   ) ______________________________

E-mail ______________________________

Date ____________ From ____________ To ____________

Emergency Contact Information

Name ______________________________

Phone (   ) ______________________________

Name ______________________________

Phone (   ) ______________________________

Name ______________________________

Phone (   ) ______________________________

My Personal Medical Journal
Published by Life Cycles Publishing, Inc.
P.O. Box 3556
Fremont, CA 94539-0355
(888) 338.0103

Designed by Gloria Lopez Cordle
Interior Graphics by Debra Pettit
Covers by Carolyn Bernal
Edited by Gloria Lopez Cordle, Debra Pettit, Carolyn Bernal
Production and Printing by Xlibris

Pictures are property of Bigstock Photo, iStock Photo, and Life Cycles Publishing, Inc.
A License Agreement was obtained for the use of all pictures by Life Cycles Publishing, Inc.

Library of Congress Control Number: 2010915939

ISBN:		
	Hard-cover	978-1-4568-0321-6
	Soft-cover	978-1-4568-0320-9
	E-book	978-1-4568-0322-3

This Book was printed by Xlibris in the United States of America.
Xlibris Corporation

82111

Acknowledgements

A special thank you.

To my children,
they gave me the inspiration
to document their medical records
in order to be an active participant in
their medical care and well being.

To my mother, Ann Lopez,
she gave me the knowledge needed
to assist her during the different stages
of her life, including
the physical challenges in her later years.
She provided the strength, poise, and
personal self reliance to maintain
a full, healthy life with her family
and friends at her side.
Her smile would light a room
and bring warmth to those she touched.
Thank you Mom,
you made a positive influence to me and
to those touched by your presence.

ꙮ

Gloria Ann Lopez

My Personal Medical Journal

Gloria Ann Lopez

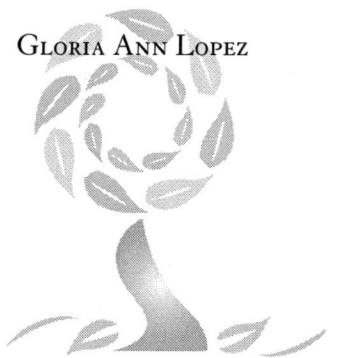

Empowerment

Today...
I feel wisdom.
I take charge of my health.
Each health provider has a piece
of my medical history.
I am the central knowledge
of what has occurred.
I work as a team member
with my professional health providers.
I feel stronger knowing
I continue to have knowledge.
I no longer have to worry
about remembering every detail of my health.
I know I have the ability to save my life
if I am unable to speak for myself.
I know I can save the life of my loved ones.
I understand by maintaining my personal or
my loved one's health record gives me empowerment.
I start by summarizing my past
and current health events, then to document each event.

I now have the peace of mind.

ꟙ

Gloria Ann Lopez

Contents

1. PERSONAL MEDICAL SUMMARY – START HERE

(You can use a form similar to the one the Doctor's office uses at your initial visit or you can obtain a Personal Medical Summary by going to www.LCPBooks.com.)

- Summarize your past and current health information.
- If you are unable to recall the exact date, use the approximate year.
- Surgeries or Procedures – If you do not remember the exact name of the surgery or procedure, give a brief explanation.
- Complete as much information you can remember, and feel free to add to it at any time.
- Make copies of your summary to keep in your files.
- Give a copy of the summary to your medical provider at EVERY visit to insure they have the current information, even if they have your computerized medical history. The medical team needs your assistance to insure the information they have is current and quickly available to provide a more effective treatment plan.

2. MY PERSONAL MEDICAL JOURNAL – START TODAY

- Transfer the important information into your new journal from your Personal Medical Summary or other notes.
- Examples:
  - Allergies to medications, foods, environmental, etc.
  - Hospitalizations / Procedures
  - Medical History – complete
  - Immunizations
  - Any other information you want to be included in your journal.
- Take your journal with you for all your medical, dental or therapy visits.

3. EMERGENCY CARD - *Located in the back of the book*

- Complete, cut out, and place in your wallet.

Note: You can customize "My Personal Medical Journal" for your individual needs.

Congratulations for taking control of your health care records!

How To Manage Your Medical History

My Personal Medical Journal has proven to be an invaluable lifesaver. It will assist you by managing your own health history, that of a child or another individual throughout his or her life. You will find this particularly useful when you go to the doctor's office or if you have a serious medical situation. Take this journal with you, especially while you are traveling and away from home, in case you require medical treatment. It will provide an overview of your medical history to assist the medical professional.

Sectioned into various categories, *My Personal Medical Journal* is a notebook to help you at an appointment with a physician, dentist, therapist, hospital, or any service agency. You can customize *My Personal Medical Journal* for your personal needs, or an individual you are caring for, by taking notes and adding your own style. This is YOUR journal and the format presented is to assist you.

To aid you further with your health management, ask your physician, dentist, and any medical professional you visit for a copy of their report for your files. This can include the following: copies of any x-rays, laboratory studies, special procedures, surgical, and special testing reports. Add any information that you feel is pertinent to you and, or will be helpful to another physician, therapist or a service provider.

For your convenience, there is an emergency card in the back of this book to fill out and keep in your wallet.

Purchase dividers and a 3 ring binder from your local supermarket, office supply store, or pharmacy, to create your Personal Health Care binder. It will make it easier for you to locate information by using dividers sectioned into the different disciplines or fields of service from which you are working. (i.e., Neurosurgery, Surgical Reports, X-ray Reports, Psychological Reports, Physician Summaries, Laboratory Results/Reports, etc.)

I suggest that you request copies of your X-ray films (i.e., an actual film copy) for your permanent health records. They will be useful as a comparison and also provide the necessary information needed for treatment. It can prove to be invaluable. To store these copies, you will find that they fit perfectly into an art portfolio that is available at your local art supply store.

You may also want a copy of your X-rays in a different format. Ask your medical facility the formats they have available (i.e., photo printout, USB flash drive, DVD, etc.) to make it easy for you to carry and store. Find out what is compatible with your computer, and the computer at the medical facility requesting a copy. It is beneficial that you have your pertinent information with you when visiting various doctors and also when traveling.

If you are an individual with special-needs and require caregivers, produce a video showing required assistance. Be sure to include feeding, bathing, cooking, transfer techniques, and personal care. This gives security to you and the caregiver knowing how best to provide the needed care.

Explain in the video:

- Daily care, showing where items need to be located in the kitchen, bathroom, and the rest of the house.
- All supplies, medical and any special items, show them and discuss what they are and how to use them, expressing any areas of concern that require specific attention.
- Instructions that are crucial to your situation, which may include incontinence and wound care, or specific attention with frequency as needed.
- Describe the medical condition, by showing literature, illustrations, or the x-ray films (if they are available) by taping them to a window that is allowing light to filter through it.
- How to use any equipment, and the maintenance required. Describe in detail how to do transfers from one piece of equipment to another, or into or out of other furnishings, when at home or when out in the community, including when traveling.
- Mobility and transportation; how to transport, local services available, how to be secured while being transported and equipment used (i.e., wheel chairs, walkers, etc.), circumstances for special consideration, and equipment for daily and long distance trips, and air travel (i.e., breakdown and securing equipment, and how to use lifts and ramps, etc.).
- Traveling; show what supplies to use, necessary equipment and how to be cared for while away from home.

This video recording will help to provide a continuum of care to enhance your quality of life. Furthering the feeling of security that you will be taken care of if your main caregiver is no longer available. My upcoming book for caregivers to assist a person with long-term care needs and maintain stabilized medical care is coming soon.

Consider your journal as a tool to assist you. There will no longer be a need to memorize every detail regarding your medical history, helping to eliminate the redundancy of information. The health care professional is pleased to know that you have your information organized. This will help to contribute to your optimum care.

Congratulations!
You now have the comfort of self-reliance and accuracy with your medical history.
Enjoy the peace of mind!

ꟿ

GLORIA ANN LOPEZ

General Overview

QUESTIONS TO ASK YOUR DOCTOR

This section will help you compile a list of questions and concerns that you will want to ask and inform your doctor at the time of your appointment.

PERSONAL INFORMATION

This overview is to assist you with general questions asked. State any diagnosis or any corrective procedure that has occurred during your lifetime.

ALERTS * CONCERNS

Maintain a log for easy recall and review.

Write any health and medical concerns that occur including areas that need to be continually observed.

MEDICATIONS

Maintain a log for easy recall and review.

Maintain all information on the medications you are taking. Ask the pharmacist to prepare a bubble pack if there are several pill-form medications taken daily. If this is not available through your local pharmacy, then purchase a weekly Sunday through Saturday plastic container (some pharmacies will give these away at no additional cost, so ask your pharmacist). Purchase a minimum of 3 to 4 boxes in different sizes and colors to identify the time of daily scheduled medication.

Place the medication in the appropriate box organized by the time of day. Check with the physician or pharmacist regarding information on which pills can or cannot be taken at the same time.

- i.e., morning, noon, dinner, evening/bedtime, other (if applicable) such as aspirin type, sleeping pills, etc.

ALLERGIES — MEDICATION * FOODS * OTHER — *Critical Section

Maintain a log for easy recall and review.

Be sure to write down any allergic reactions, and what medication or treatment was necessary to resolve this problem. This is extremely vital for any medical professional who is assisting you.

HOSPITALIZATIONS * SURGERIES * PROCEDURES

Maintain a log for easy recall and review.

It is beneficial that you, the physician, or the dentist, summarize the procedure, complications, and any notes in this area. Ask for a copy of the Doctor's surgical or procedure notes for your file or binder.

MEDICAL * DOCTOR APPOINTMENTS

Maintain a log for easy recall and review

Write down the reason for the visit, specify if it is routine or an emergency, etc. This is especially helpful to keep abreast of what has occurred, and for a continuum of health. You can have the doctor summarize the procedure, complications, and any notes in this area. If, you consider this information beneficial, ask for a copy of the doctor's report for your file or binder.

DENTAL APPOINTMENTS

Maintain a log for easy recall and review

Write down the reason for the visit, specify if it is routine or an emergency, etc. This is especially helpful to keep abreast of what has occurred, and for a continuum of health. You can have the dentist summarize the procedure, complications, and any notes in this area. If, you consider this information beneficial, ask for a copy of the doctor's report for your file or binder.

LABORATORY WORK * X-RAY

Maintain a log for easy recall and review

State the type of test, the reason for it and the results. For your Personal Health Care binder, you may want to request a copy of the report and, or x-rays, depending on the test. This is useful especially for future reference and to assist any professional when evaluating a medical treatment or condition. If the service provider will not release the report to you, then request that it be sent to your physician so that you can obtain a copy.

IMMUNIZATIONS * INJECTIONS

Maintain a log for easy recall and review

These records will be needed throughout your lifetime.

SERVICE AGENCIES

This information is helpful when utilizing services from a particular program, association or provider. (i.e., funding sources, physical therapy, nutritionist, transportation, educational programs, etc.)

NAMES AND ADDRESS INDEX

Keep the phone numbers and addresses of any one who is assisting you with your medical and dental health care.

EMERGENCY CARD

Fill in the information on the card, cut it out, fold it and put it in your wallet.

<u>Note</u>: You can customize "My Personal Medical Journal" for your individual needs.

YOU HAVE THE RIGHT TO ASK YOUR DOCTOR QUESTIONS

Leave Your Comfort Zone and Speak Up

Asking questions will help you establish communication with your doctor and begin the process of forming a partnership with your medical professionals.

IMPORTANT QUESTIONS TO ASK YOUR DOCTOR

This list consists of 5 IMPORTANT CATEGORIES, each having a list of questions. You can use this information as a guide to develop your personal list of questions pertaining to your medical concerns.

1. Illness, Symptoms and Clarity
2. Medication
3. Tests and Procedures
4. Copy of All Reports
5. Documentation

ILLNESS, SYMPTOMS AND CLARITY

It is very important before going to your doctor visit, to write a list of questions concerning your symptoms and health concerns. If you did not have a chance to write them down, take the opportunity while you are waiting at the reception area or the doctor's exam room. Make sure you ask for clarity if you do not understand the answer given by the medical professional.

1. Describe ALL your symptoms.
2. Ask what is causing you to feel ill?
3. Be sure to ask for clarity if you do not understand.
4. Ask the doctor for written material concerning the medical condition, or to draw a picture to describe the area affected. It is vital that you know what is happening and why.
5. Ask how serious is your condition, and, how long will it take to get better.
6. Ask what should be avoided that will prevent or slow your healing process. (i.e., activities, household chores, lifting limitations, foods, prescribed or over-the-counter medications and dietary supplements).

MEDICATION

At the time of your appointment, it is best to remind your doctor of all current medications. Your medical providers may have a file with your medical history right in front of them. It is possible they did not have time to review it. You need to remind them and advocate for yourself. **Make sure to bring a list of *all the medications and supplements* you are currently taking.**

- **Prescription**
- **Over-the-counter**
- **Herbal or Dietary Supplements**
- **Mail-order**

You may want to take the actual items with you to the doctor. It is also suggested that you follow the same procedure with your pharmacist. This will help to avoid any conflict or allergic reaction that might be caused by the combination of old and new medications.

There might come a time when you see a different doctor, so it is crucial you have this information documented. The medical provider needs to be aware of the allergies you have that include food and any medical or herbal supplements.

Be sure to ask your doctor and pharmacist;

1. What will this medication do and how long should it be taken?
2. Are there any allergic reactions or side effects and what should be expected? (If you receive a printout make sure to read it.)
3. How will the new prescription react with other medications and dietary supplements currently taken?

EMERGENCY ROOM

If you have to go to the Emergency Room or be admitted to the hospital, not everyone is aware of your medical history. You may find that you need to write down your allergies towards medications, latex, etc., in large letters on a large blank sheet of paper and tape it to the wall. Place it where it is easily seen by the medical staff. This will be particularly useful for you and those caring for you.

TEST, PROCEDURES, SURGERIES AND RESULTS

Document the results of a TEST, a PROCEDURE or a SURGERY, and if needed, ask your medical professional for permission to tape record the explanation of your condition, and how you are to proceed. Reassure them that this is for you and your family's personal understanding. IT IS NOT FOR LEGAL PURPOSES.

1. Ask what is the purpose of the TEST, PROCEDURE or SURGERY?
2. Why is this TEST needed?
3. Ask about side effects and what should be expected. (i.e., Are there any type of limitations and for how long; will assistance be needed for driving or at home, etc.)
4. Are there any reactions to foods and allergies? (i.e., If you have allergies to seafood, then an iodine test might be a problem.)

5. Make sure you find out what are the risks. Ask if it is going to hurt and if there is anything to ease the pain. Remember all questions are vital to your well being.
6. Ask where the PROCEDURE or SURGERY will be performed; the doctor's office, a specific lab or another medical facility? Be sure to find out what preparations and post care is needed.
7. Find out how much the procedure and surgery cost and what are the payment expectations. Does your insurance cover the cost?

In addition, you may want to have a person of confidence go along with you to an appointment. They can help you in documenting the information given by your medical professional, and be available for assisting with your needs and transportation.

COPY OF ALL REPORTS

Make sure you ask your medical professional for copies of all your medical reports; x-rays, lab reports, office visits, and any surgical procedures. When seeing other medical providers you will find that this information will be vital at some point in time. (refer to "How to Manage your Medical History" pages 12-13)

DOCUMENTATION

Maintaining a record of your **Personal Health Information** is beneficial to you and your family's well being. Remember you are ultimately responsible for making decisions concerning your health. The information that you document should be accurate, reliable, and complete. This will give you control over how your health information is accessed, used, and disclosed.

By documenting your personal health information it becomes a tool you can use to collect, tract and share past and current information about you and your family's health. Providing your medical and health care professionals more insight into your personal health history helps to save you money, and possibly, one day, your life.

START TODAY by keeping a complete record of your *personal health history* in ***"My Personal Medical Journal"***.
This will help you to reduce the risk of medical mistakes and medical errors.

REMEMBER, YOU HAVE THE RIGHT TO ASK YOUR DOCTOR QUESTIONS
Leave Your Comfort Zone and Speak Up

- Do not fall under the false impression that the medical professional knows all.
- The medical providers only know what you tell them!
- You have the power to improve your medical outcome. (This will help to reduce the medical mistakes and errors that occur at an alarming percentage.)
- Remember **Your Life is in Your Own Hands.**
- You have the right to ask any question, even if it is confrontational.

That one question just might save your life!

Personal Information

This overview is to assist you with general questions asked. State any diagnosis or any corrective procedure that has occurred during your lifetime.

Personal Information

Personal Information

Name ______________________________

Address ______________________________

City ______________ State ______ Zip ______ Country ______

Phone (   ) ______________ Fax (   ) ______________

Cell (   ) ______________ E-mail ______________

DOB ______________ Religion ______________

S.S.# XXX-XX-______________ Blood Type ______________

Ethnicity ______________________________

Children ______________________________

ﷺ

Nearest Relative Name ______________________________

Relationship ______________ Phone (   ) ______________

Other Phone (   ) ______________________________

E-mail ______________________________

Family History

❑ Attach separate sheet with more information.

Date	Doctor	Phone	Specialty

Comments ______________________________

____

____

____

Physicians / Dentists

Place full address information in the Name & Address section. Obtain the business card for easy reference.

Date	Doctor	Phone	Specialty

Insurance Information

Keep a photocopy of your insurance cards for easy reference.

Medicare # ______ Medical ______

Other: Type ______ # ______

Subscriber ______

Subscriber # ______ Effective ______

Medical Insurance Carrier ______

Group # ______

Member Services Phone ( ) ______

Co-Pay $ ______ Office Visit $ ______ Hospital $ ______

ER $ ______ Rx $ ______ Other $ ______

Primary Physician ______

Plan Code ______

Employer ______

Address ______ Phone ( ) ______

Dental Carrier ______ Plan # ______

Member Services Phone ( ) ______ Co-Pay $ ______

Other Coverage ______

NOTE ______

Specific Notations

Specific Notations:

❑ **Allergies:** ❑ Latex ❑ Penicillin ❑ Iodine ❑ Metal ❑ Other: see list

❑ **Phobias:** ❑ Shots / Needles ❑ Dental ❑ Other ____________________

❑ **Reflex Notation:** ❑ Gag ❑ Other ____________________

❑ **Heart Pacemaker**

❑ **Prothesis / Implants:**

Type ❑ Dentures ❑ Fixed ❑ Removable ❑ Full ❑ Partial

❑ Body ❑ External ____________________

❑ Internal ____________________

Reference - L=Left Side R=Right Side F=Front B=Back H=Head

Example:
Enter Date, place a ☑ in correct Area of Concern, and add Explanation of Affected Area.

Date	Area of Concern	Explanation of Affected Area
	❑ L ❑ R ❑ F ❑ B ❑ H	
	❑ L ❑ R ❑ F ❑ B ❑ H	
	❑ L ❑ R ❑ F ❑ B ❑ H	
	❑ L ❑ R ❑ F ❑ B ❑ H	
	❑ L ❑ R ❑ F ❑ B ❑ H	
	❑ L ❑ R ❑ F ❑ B ❑ H	
	❑ L ❑ R ❑ F ❑ B ❑ H	

Diagnosis

Maintain a log for easy recall and review.

Date	Diagnosis	Explanation	Resolved

Additional Notes____________________________________

Today's Blessing

Today is a new blessing.
One filled with
promise,
joy,
understanding,
listening,
and learning.
One filled with those surrounding us,
and with a gift of a gentle smile.
Take this day and give thanks for each
blessing that unfolds,
for it is a gift to cherish.

ഇ

Gloria Ann Lopez

Alerts * Concerns

Alerts * Concerns

Log

Maintain a log for easy recall and review.

Alerts and Concerns

Write any health and medical concerns that occur, including areas that need to be continually observed.

Notes

Alerts * Concerns

Alerts * Concerns Log

Maintain a log for easy recall and review.

Date	Condition	Concern

Alerts * Concerns

Alerts * Concerns

Write any health and medical concerns that occur including areas that need to be continually observed.

Date ____________ Dr. / Other ____________

Condition / Diagnosis ____________

____

Lab ❑ X-ray ❑ Other Tests ____________

Next Appointment Date ____________ Time ____________

Describe ____________

____

____

Date ____________ Dr. / Other ____________

Condition / Diagnosis ____________

____

❑ Lab ❑ X-ray ❑ Other Tests ____________

Next Appointment Date ____________ Time ____________

Describe ____________

____

____

Date ____________ Dr. / Other ____________

Condition / Diagnosis ____________

____

❑ Lab ❑ X-ray ❑ Other Tests ____________

Next Appointment Date ____________ Time ____________

Describe ____________

____

____

Alerts * Concerns

Write any health and medical concerns that occur including areas that need to be continually observed.

Date __________ Dr. / Other __________

Condition / Diagnosis __________

Lab ❑ X-ray ❑ Other Tests __________

Next Appointment Date __________ Time __________

Describe __________

Date __________ Dr. / Other __________

Condition / Diagnosis __________

❑ Lab ❑ X-ray ❑ Other Tests __________

Next Appointment Date __________ Time __________

Describe __________

Date __________ Dr. / Other __________

Condition / Diagnosis __________

❑ Lab ❑ X-ray ❑ Other Tests __________

Next Appointment Date __________ Time __________

Describe __________

Alerts * Concerns

Write any health and medical concerns that occur including areas that need to be continually observed.

Date ____________ Dr. / Other ____________

Condition / Diagnosis ____________

____

Lab ❑ X-ray ❑ Other Tests ____________

Next Appointment Date ____________ Time ____________

Describe ____________

____

____

Date ____________ Dr. / Other ____________

Condition / Diagnosis ____________

____

❑ Lab ❑ X-ray ❑ Other Tests ____________

Next Appointment Date ____________ Time ____________

Describe ____________

____

____

Date ____________ Dr. / Other ____________

Condition / Diagnosis ____________

____

❑ Lab ❑ X-ray ❑ Other Tests ____________

Next Appointment Date ____________ Time ____________

Describe ____________

____

____

Alerts * Concerns

Write any health and medical concerns that occur including areas that need to be continually observed.

Date ____________ Dr. / Other ____________

Condition / Diagnosis ____________

____

Lab ❑ X-ray ❑ Other Tests ____________

Next Appointment Date ____________ Time ____________

Describe ____________

____

____

Date ____________ Dr. / Other ____________

Condition / Diagnosis ____________

____

❑ Lab ❑ X-ray ❑ Other Tests ____________

Next Appointment Date ____________ Time ____________

Describe ____________

____

____

Date ____________ Dr. / Other ____________

Condition / Diagnosis ____________

____

❑ Lab ❑ X-ray ❑ Other Tests ____________

Next Appointment Date ____________ Time ____________

Describe ____________

____

____

Alerts * Concerns

Alerts * Concerns

Write any health and medical concerns that occur including areas that need to be continually observed.

Date ____________________ Dr. / Other ____________________

Condition / Diagnosis ____________________

____

Lab ❑ X-ray ❑ Other Tests ____________________

Next Appointment Date ____________________ Time ____________________

Describe ____________________

____

____

Date ____________________ Dr. / Other ____________________

Condition / Diagnosis ____________________

____

❑ Lab ❑ X-ray ❑ Other Tests ____________________

Next Appointment Date ____________________ Time ____________________

Describe ____________________

____

____

Date ____________________ Dr. / Other ____________________

Condition / Diagnosis ____________________

____

❑ Lab ❑ X-ray ❑ Other Tests ____________________

Next Appointment Date ____________________ Time ____________________

Describe ____________________

____

____

MEDICATIONS
LOG, RECORDS AND DAILY SCHEDULE

Log

It is important to keep a record of all your prescriptions, including over-the-counter, herbal or dietary supplements and mail order medications to assist medical professionals.

Records

Maintain the information and Doctor's orders on the medications you are taking.

Daily Schedule

Maintain all information on the medications you are taking. Space is provided to document what medications are taken each day of the week. Place the medication in the appropriate box organized by the time of day. Check with the physician or pharmacist regarding information on which pills can or cannot be taken at the same time.

Ask the pharmacist to prepare a bubble pack if there are several pill-form medications taken daily. If this is not available through your local pharmacy, then purchase a weekly Sunday through Saturday plastic container (some pharmacies will give these away at no additional cost, so ask your pharmacist). Purchase a minimum of 3 to 4 boxes in different sizes and colors to identify the time of daily medication scheduled.

Notes

Medications

Medication Log

Maintain a log/list on your medications for easy access.

Place a: (✓) or **date** in Reaction when symptoms occur then explain in Allergy Section - Medication.

(✓) or **date** at the *Stopped* Section when finished taking your medication.

DATE	DRUG or APPLICATION	DOSAGE	FREQUENCY	REACTION *See Allergy Section	STOPPED/DISCONTINUED	COMMENTS

Medications

Medication Log

Maintain a log/list on your medications for easy access.

Place a: (✓) or **date** in Reaction when symptoms occur then explain in Allergy Section - Medication.

(✓) or **date** at the *Stopped* Section when finished taking your medication.

DATE	DRUG or APPLICATION	DOSAGE	FREQUENCY	REACTION *See Allergy Section	STOPPED/DISCONTINUED	COMMENTS

Medications

Medication Log

Maintain a log/list on your medications for easy access.

Place a: (✓) or **date** in Reaction when symptoms occur then explain in Allergy Section - Medication.

(✓) or **date** at the *Stopped* Section when finished taking your medication.

DATE	DRUG or APPLICATION	DOSAGE	FREQUENCY	REACTION *See Allergy Section	STOPPED/DISCONTINUED	COMMENTS

Medications

Medication Log

Maintain a log/list on your medications for easy access.

Place a: (✓) or **date** in Reaction when symptoms occur then explain in Allergy Section - Medication.

(✓) or **date** at the *Stopped* Section when finished taking your medication.

DATE	DRUG or APPLICATION	DOSAGE	FREQUENCY	REACTION *See Allergy Section	STOPPED/DISCONTINUED	COMMENTS

Medication Records

Date ______________ Dr. ________________________________ Phone ( ) ______________

Medication ____ Rx # ______________

Purpose ____

Dosage __________ mg _____ Length *(days)* ____________ Other ______________

Time

				Other

Special instructions *(i.e., taken with food, increase water, etc.)* ______________

____

Side effects (i.e., may cause drowsiness, etc.) ______________________________

____

Discontinued Date ______________________ ❑ Monthly prescription refill

Reason: ❑ Completed ❑ Reaction: *Be sure to add to Allergy Section - Medication.*

Date ______________ Dr. ________________________________ Phone ( ) ______________

Medication ____ Rx # ______________

Purpose ____

Dosage __________ mg _____ Length *(days)* ____________ Other ______________

Time

				Other

Special instructions *(i.e., taken with food, increase water, etc.)* ______________

____

Side effects (i.e., may cause drowsiness, etc.) ______________________________

____

Discontinued Date ______________________ ❑ Monthly prescription refill

Reason: ❑ Completed ❑ Reaction: *Be sure to add to Allergy Section - Medication.*

Date ______________ Dr. ________________________________ Phone ( ) ______________

Medication ____ Rx # ______________

Purpose ____

Dosage __________ mg _____ Length *(days)* ____________ Other ______________

Time

				Other

Special instructions *(i.e., taken with food, increase water, etc.)* ______________

____

Side effects (i.e., may cause drowsiness, etc.) ______________________________

____

Discontinued Date ______________________ ❑ Monthly prescription refill

Reason: ❑ Completed ❑ Reaction: *Be sure to add to Allergy Section - Medication.*

Medication Records

Date ______________ Dr. __________________________________ Phone (   ) ______________

Medication ____ Rx # ______________________

Purpose ____

Dosage ____________ mg _____ Length *(days)* ______________ Other ______________

Time

				Other

Special instructions *(i.e., taken with food, increase water, etc.)* ______________________

____

Side effects (i.e., may cause drowsiness, etc.) ______________________________

____

Discontinued Date ________________________ ❑ Monthly prescription refill

Reason: ❑ Completed ❑ Reaction: *Be sure to add to Allergy Section - Medication.*

Date ______________ Dr. __________________________________ Phone (   ) ______________

Medication ____ Rx # ______________________

Purpose ____

Dosage ____________ mg _____ Length *(days)* ______________ Other ______________

Time

				Other

Special instructions *(i.e., taken with food, increase water, etc.)* ______________________

____

Side effects (i.e., may cause drowsiness, etc.) ______________________________

____

Discontinued Date ________________________ ❑ Monthly prescription refill

Reason: ❑ Completed ❑ Reaction: *Be sure to add to Allergy Section - Medication.*

Date ______________ Dr. __________________________________ Phone (   ) ______________

Medication ____ Rx # ______________________

Purpose ____

Dosage ____________ mg _____ Length *(days)* ______________ Other ______________

Time

				Other

Special instructions *(i.e., taken with food, increase water, etc.)* ______________________

____

Side effects (i.e., may cause drowsiness, etc.) ______________________________

____

Discontinued Date ________________________ ❑ Monthly prescription refill

Reason: ❑ Completed ❑ Reaction: *Be sure to add to Allergy Section - Medication.*

Medication Records

Date ______________ Dr. __________________________________ Phone (______) ______________

Medication ____ Rx # ______________________

Purpose ____

Dosage ____________ mg _____ Length *(days)* ______________ Other ______________________

Time

				Other

Special instructions *(i.e., taken with food, increase water, etc.)* ______________________

____

Side effects (i.e., may cause drowsiness, etc.) ____

____

Discontinued Date ________________________ ❑ Monthly prescription refill

Reason: ❑ Completed ❑ Reaction: *Be sure to add to Allergy Section - Medication.*

Date ______________ Dr. __________________________________ Phone (______) ______________

Medication ____ Rx # ______________________

Purpose ____

Dosage ____________ mg _____ Length *(days)* ______________ Other ______________________

Time

				Other

Special instructions *(i.e., taken with food, increase water, etc.)* ______________________

____

Side effects (i.e., may cause drowsiness, etc.) ____

____

Discontinued Date ________________________ ❑ Monthly prescription refill

Reason: ❑ Completed ❑ Reaction: *Be sure to add to Allergy Section - Medication.*

Date ______________ Dr. __________________________________ Phone (______) ______________

Medication ____ Rx # ______________________

Purpose ____

Dosage ____________ mg _____ Length *(days)* ______________ Other ______________________

Time

				Other

Special instructions *(i.e., taken with food, increase water, etc.)* ______________________

____

Side effects (i.e., may cause drowsiness, etc.) ____

____

Discontinued Date ________________________ ❑ Monthly prescription refill

Reason: ❑ Completed ❑ Reaction: *Be sure to add to Allergy Section - Medication.*

Medication Records

Date ______________ Dr. ______________________________ Phone (   ) ______________

Medication ______________________________ Rx # ______________

Purpose ____

Dosage __________ mg _____ Length *(days)* __________ Other ______________

Time

				Other

Special instructions *(i.e., taken with food, increase water, etc.)* ______________

____

Side effects (i.e., may cause drowsiness, etc.) ______________

____

Discontinued Date ______________ ❑ Monthly prescription refill

Reason: ❑ Completed ❑ Reaction: *Be sure to add to Allergy Section - Medication.*

Date ______________ Dr. ______________________________ Phone (   ) ______________

Medication ______________________________ Rx # ______________

Purpose ____

Dosage __________ mg _____ Length *(days)* __________ Other ______________

Time

				Other

Special instructions *(i.e., taken with food, increase water, etc.)* ______________

____

Side effects (i.e., may cause drowsiness, etc.) ______________

____

Discontinued Date ______________ ❑ Monthly prescription refill

Reason: ❑ Completed ❑ Reaction: *Be sure to add to Allergy Section - Medication.*

Date ______________ Dr. ______________________________ Phone (   ) ______________

Medication ______________________________ Rx # ______________

Purpose ____

Dosage __________ mg _____ Length *(days)* __________ Other ______________

Time

				Other

Special instructions *(i.e., taken with food, increase water, etc.)* ______________

____

Side effects (i.e., may cause drowsiness, etc.) ______________

____

Discontinued Date ______________ ❑ Monthly prescription refill

Reason: ❑ Completed ❑ Reaction: *Be sure to add to Allergy Section - Medication.*

Medication Records

Date ______________ Dr. ________________________________ Phone (______) ____________

Medication ____ Rx # ____________________

Purpose ____

Dosage ____________ mg ______ Length *(days)* ______________ Other ________________

Time

				Other

Special instructions *(i.e., taken with food, increase water, etc.)* ____________________

____

Side effects (i.e., may cause drowsiness, etc.) ___________________________________

____

Discontinued Date ______________________ ❑ Monthly prescription refill

Reason: ❑ Completed ❑ Reaction: *Be sure to add to Allergy Section - Medication.*

Date ______________ Dr. ________________________________ Phone (______) ____________

Medication ____ Rx # ____________________

Purpose ____

Dosage ____________ mg ______ Length *(days)* ______________ Other ________________

Time

				Other

Special instructions *(i.e., taken with food, increase water, etc.)* ____________________

____

Side effects (i.e., may cause drowsiness, etc.) ___________________________________

____

Discontinued Date ______________________ ❑ Monthly prescription refill

Reason: ❑ Completed ❑ Reaction: *Be sure to add to Allergy Section - Medication.*

Date ______________ Dr. ________________________________ Phone (______) ____________

Medication ____ Rx # ____________________

Purpose ____

Dosage ____________ mg ______ Length *(days)* ______________ Other ________________

Time

				Other

Special instructions *(i.e., taken with food, increase water, etc.)* ____________________

____

Side effects (i.e., may cause drowsiness, etc.) ___________________________________

____

Discontinued Date ______________________ ❑ Monthly prescription refill

Reason: ❑ Completed ❑ Reaction: *Be sure to add to Allergy Section - Medication.*

Medication Records

Date ____________ Dr. ______________________________ Phone ( ) ____________

Medication ______________________________________ Rx # ____________

Purpose ____

Dosage __________ mg _____ Length *(days)* __________ Other ____________

Time

				Other

Special instructions *(i.e., taken with food, increase water, etc.)* ____________

____

Side effects (i.e., may cause drowsiness, etc.) ______________________________

____

Discontinued Date ____________________ ❑ Monthly prescription refill

Reason: ❑ Completed ❑ Reaction: *Be sure to add to Allergy Section - Medication.*

Date ____________ Dr. ______________________________ Phone ( ) ____________

Medication ______________________________________ Rx # ____________

Purpose ____

Dosage __________ mg _____ Length *(days)* __________ Other ____________

Time

				Other

Special instructions *(i.e., taken with food, increase water, etc.)* ____________

____

Side effects (i.e., may cause drowsiness, etc.) ______________________________

____

Discontinued Date ____________________ ❑ Monthly prescription refill

Reason: ❑ Completed ❑ Reaction: *Be sure to add to Allergy Section - Medication.*

Date ____________ Dr. ______________________________ Phone ( ) ____________

Medication ______________________________________ Rx # ____________

Purpose ____

Dosage __________ mg _____ Length *(days)* __________ Other ____________

Time

				Other

Special instructions *(i.e., taken with food, increase water, etc.)* ____________

____

Side effects (i.e., may cause drowsiness, etc.) ______________________________

____

Discontinued Date ____________________ ❑ Monthly prescription refill

Reason: ❑ Completed ❑ Reaction: *Be sure to add to Allergy Section - Medication.*

Medication Records

Date ______________ Dr. ________________________________ Phone ( ) ____________

Medication ____ Rx # ____________________

Purpose ____

Dosage ____________ mg _____ Length *(days)* ____________ Other ______________

Time

				Other

Special instructions *(i.e., taken with food, increase water, etc.)* ________________

____

Side effects (i.e., may cause drowsiness, etc.) __________________________

____

Discontinued Date ______________________ ❑ Monthly prescription refill

Reason: ❑ Completed ❑ Reaction: *Be sure to add to Allergy Section - Medication.*

Date ______________ Dr. ________________________________ Phone ( ) ____________

Medication ____ Rx # ____________________

Purpose ____

Dosage ____________ mg _____ Length *(days)* ____________ Other ______________

Time

				Other

Special instructions *(i.e., taken with food, increase water, etc.)* ________________

____

Side effects (i.e., may cause drowsiness, etc.) __________________________

____

Discontinued Date ______________________ ❑ Monthly prescription refill

Reason: ❑ Completed ❑ Reaction: *Be sure to add to Allergy Section - Medication.*

Date ______________ Dr. ________________________________ Phone ( ) ____________

Medication ____ Rx # ____________________

Purpose ____

Dosage ____________ mg _____ Length *(days)* ____________ Other ______________

Time

				Other

Special instructions *(i.e., taken with food, increase water, etc.)* ________________

____

Side effects (i.e., may cause drowsiness, etc.) __________________________

____

Discontinued Date ______________________ ❑ Monthly prescription refill

Reason: ❑ Completed ❑ Reaction: *Be sure to add to Allergy Section - Medication.*

Medication Records

Date ____________ Dr. ______________________________ Phone (   ) ______________

Medication ______________________________________ Rx # ______________

Purpose ____

Dosage __________ mg _____ Length *(days)* __________ Other ______________

Time

				Other

Special instructions *(i.e., taken with food, increase water, etc.)* ______________

____

Side effects (i.e., may cause drowsiness, etc.) ______________________________

____

Discontinued Date ______________ ❑ Monthly prescription refill

Reason: ❑ Completed ❑ Reaction: *Be sure to add to Allergy Section - Medication.*

Date ____________ Dr. ______________________________ Phone (   ) ______________

Medication ______________________________________ Rx # ______________

Purpose ____

Dosage __________ mg _____ Length *(days)* __________ Other ______________

Time

				Other

Special instructions *(i.e., taken with food, increase water, etc.)* ______________

____

Side effects (i.e., may cause drowsiness, etc.) ______________________________

____

Discontinued Date ______________ ❑ Monthly prescription refill

Reason: ❑ Completed ❑ Reaction: *Be sure to add to Allergy Section - Medication.*

Date ____________ Dr. ______________________________ Phone (   ) ______________

Medication ______________________________________ Rx # ______________

Purpose ____

Dosage __________ mg _____ Length *(days)* __________ Other ______________

Time

				Other

Special instructions *(i.e., taken with food, increase water, etc.)* ______________

____

Side effects (i.e., may cause drowsiness, etc.) ______________________________

____

Discontinued Date ______________ ❑ Monthly prescription refill

Reason: ❑ Completed ❑ Reaction: *Be sure to add to Allergy Section - Medication.*

Medication Records

Date ____________ Dr. ____________________________ Phone ( ) ____________

Medication ____________________________________ Rx # ____________

Purpose ____

Dosage ________ mg _____ Length *(days)* __________ Other ____________

Time

				Other

Special instructions *(i.e., taken with food, increase water, etc.)* ____________

____

Side effects (i.e., may cause drowsiness, etc.) ____________________

____

Discontinued Date ____________ ❑ Monthly prescription refill

Reason: ❑ Completed ❑ Reaction: *Be sure to add to Allergy Section - Medication.*

Date ____________ Dr. ____________________________ Phone ( ) ____________

Medication ____________________________________ Rx # ____________

Purpose ____

Dosage ________ mg _____ Length *(days)* __________ Other ____________

Time

				Other

Special instructions *(i.e., taken with food, increase water, etc.)* ____________

____

Side effects (i.e., may cause drowsiness, etc.) ____________________

____

Discontinued Date ____________ ❑ Monthly prescription refill

Reason: ❑ Completed ❑ Reaction: *Be sure to add to Allergy Section - Medication.*

Date ____________ Dr. ____________________________ Phone ( ) ____________

Medication ____________________________________ Rx # ____________

Purpose ____

Dosage ________ mg _____ Length *(days)* __________ Other ____________

Time

				Other

Special instructions *(i.e., taken with food, increase water, etc.)* ____________

____

Side effects (i.e., may cause drowsiness, etc.) ____________________

____

Discontinued Date ____________ ❑ Monthly prescription refill

Reason: ❑ Completed ❑ Reaction: *Be sure to add to Allergy Section - Medication.*

Medication Records

Date ______________ Dr. ________________________________ Phone ( ) ______________

Medication ____ Rx # ______________

Purpose ____

Dosage ____________ mg _____ Length *(days)* ______________ Other ______________

Time

				Other

Special instructions *(i.e., taken with food, increase water, etc.)* ______________________

____

Side effects (i.e., may cause drowsiness, etc.) ______________________________

____

Discontinued Date ______________________ ❑ Monthly prescription refill

Reason: ❑ Completed ❑ Reaction: *Be sure to add to Allergy Section - Medication.*

Date ______________ Dr. ________________________________ Phone ( ) ______________

Medication ____ Rx # ______________

Purpose ____

Dosage ____________ mg _____ Length *(days)* ______________ Other ______________

Time

				Other

Special instructions *(i.e., taken with food, increase water, etc.)* ______________________

____

Side effects (i.e., may cause drowsiness, etc.) ______________________________

____

Discontinued Date ______________________ ❑ Monthly prescription refill

Reason: ❑ Completed ❑ Reaction: *Be sure to add to Allergy Section - Medication.*

Date ______________ Dr. ________________________________ Phone ( ) ______________

Medication ____ Rx # ______________

Purpose ____

Dosage ____________ mg _____ Length *(days)* ______________ Other ______________

Time

				Other

Special instructions *(i.e., taken with food, increase water, etc.)* ______________________

____

Side effects (i.e., may cause drowsiness, etc.) ______________________________

____

Discontinued Date ______________________ ❑ Monthly prescription refill

Reason: ❑ Completed ❑ Reaction: *Be sure to add to Allergy Section - Medication.*

Medication Records

Date ____________ Dr. ____________________________ Phone (   ) ____________

Medication ____________________________________ Rx # ____________

Purpose ____

Dosage ________ mg _____ Length *(days)* ________ Other ____________

Time				*Other*

Special instructions *(i.e., taken with food, increase water, etc.)* ____________

____

Side effects (i.e., may cause drowsiness, etc.) ____________

____

Discontinued Date ____________ ❑ Monthly prescription refill

Reason: ❑ Completed ❑ Reaction: *Be sure to add to Allergy Section - Medication.*

Date ____________ Dr. ____________________________ Phone (   ) ____________

Medication ____________________________________ Rx # ____________

Purpose ____

Dosage ________ mg _____ Length *(days)* ________ Other ____________

Time				*Other*

Special instructions *(i.e., taken with food, increase water, etc.)* ____________

____

Side effects (i.e., may cause drowsiness, etc.) ____________

____

Discontinued Date ____________ ❑ Monthly prescription refill

Reason: ❑ Completed ❑ Reaction: *Be sure to add to Allergy Section - Medication.*

Date ____________ Dr. ____________________________ Phone (   ) ____________

Medication ____________________________________ Rx # ____________

Purpose ____

Dosage ________ mg _____ Length *(days)* ________ Other ____________

Time				*Other*

Special instructions *(i.e., taken with food, increase water, etc.)* ____________

____

Side effects (i.e., may cause drowsiness, etc.) ____________

____

Discontinued Date ____________ ❑ Monthly prescription refill

Reason: ❑ Completed ❑ Reaction: *Be sure to add to Allergy Section - Medication.*

Medication Records

Date ______________ Dr. ________________________________ Phone (   ) ______________

Medication ____ Rx # ______________

Purpose ____

Dosage ____________ mg _____ Length *(days)* ____________ Other ______________

Time

				Other

Special instructions *(i.e., taken with food, increase water, etc.)* ______________________

____

Side effects (i.e., may cause drowsiness, etc.) ______________________________

____

Discontinued Date ______________________ ❑ Monthly prescription refill

Reason: ❑ Completed ❑ Reaction: *Be sure to add to Allergy Section - Medication.*

Date ______________ Dr. ________________________________ Phone (   ) ______________

Medication ____ Rx # ______________

Purpose ____

Dosage ____________ mg _____ Length *(days)* ____________ Other ______________

Time

				Other

Special instructions *(i.e., taken with food, increase water, etc.)* ______________________

____

Side effects (i.e., may cause drowsiness, etc.) ______________________________

____

Discontinued Date ______________________ ❑ Monthly prescription refill

Reason: ❑ Completed ❑ Reaction: *Be sure to add to Allergy Section - Medication.*

Date ______________ Dr. ________________________________ Phone (   ) ______________

Medication ____ Rx # ______________

Purpose ____

Dosage ____________ mg _____ Length *(days)* ____________ Other ______________

Time

				Other

Special instructions *(i.e., taken with food, increase water, etc.)* ______________________

____

Side effects (i.e., may cause drowsiness, etc.) ______________________________

____

Discontinued Date ______________________ ❑ Monthly prescription refill

Reason: ❑ Completed ❑ Reaction: *Be sure to add to Allergy Section - Medication.*

Medication Records

Date ______________ Dr. ________________________________ Phone (   ) ______________

Medication ____ Rx # ______________

Purpose ____

Dosage ____________ mg _____ Length *(days)* ______________ Other ______________

Time

				Other

Special instructions *(i.e., taken with food, increase water, etc.)* ________________________

____

Side effects (i.e., may cause drowsiness, etc.) ________________________________

____

Discontinued Date ______________________ ❑ Monthly prescription refill

Reason: ❑ Completed ❑ Reaction: *Be sure to add to Allergy Section - Medication.*

Date ______________ Dr. ________________________________ Phone (   ) ______________

Medication ____ Rx # ______________

Purpose ____

Dosage ____________ mg _____ Length *(days)* ______________ Other ______________

Time

				Other

Special instructions *(i.e., taken with food, increase water, etc.)* ________________________

____

Side effects (i.e., may cause drowsiness, etc.) ________________________________

____

Discontinued Date ______________________ ❑ Monthly prescription refill

Reason: ❑ Completed ❑ Reaction: *Be sure to add to Allergy Section - Medication.*

Date ______________ Dr. ________________________________ Phone (   ) ______________

Medication ____ Rx # ______________

Purpose ____

Dosage ____________ mg _____ Length *(days)* ______________ Other ______________

Time

				Other

Special instructions *(i.e., taken with food, increase water, etc.)* ________________________

____

Side effects (i.e., may cause drowsiness, etc.) ________________________________

____

Discontinued Date ______________________ ❑ Monthly prescription refill

Reason: ❑ Completed ❑ Reaction: *Be sure to add to Allergy Section - Medication.*

Medication Records

Date ______________ Dr. ______________________________ Phone ( ) ______________

Medication ______________________________________ Rx # ______________

Purpose ____

Dosage __________ mg _____ Length *(days)* __________ Other __________

Time

				Other

Special instructions *(i.e., taken with food, increase water, etc.)* ______________

____

Side effects (i.e., may cause drowsiness, etc.) ______________________________

____

Discontinued Date ______________ ❑ Monthly prescription refill

Reason: ❑ Completed ❑ Reaction: *Be sure to add to Allergy Section - Medication.*

Date ______________ Dr. ______________________________ Phone ( ) ______________

Medication ______________________________________ Rx # ______________

Purpose ____

Dosage __________ mg _____ Length *(days)* __________ Other __________

Time

				Other

Special instructions *(i.e., taken with food, increase water, etc.)* ______________

____

Side effects (i.e., may cause drowsiness, etc.) ______________________________

____

Discontinued Date ______________ ❑ Monthly prescription refill

Reason: ❑ Completed ❑ Reaction: *Be sure to add to Allergy Section - Medication.*

Date ______________ Dr. ______________________________ Phone ( ) ______________

Medication ______________________________________ Rx # ______________

Purpose ____

Dosage __________ mg _____ Length *(days)* __________ Other __________

Time

				Other

Special instructions *(i.e., taken with food, increase water, etc.)* ______________

____

Side effects (i.e., may cause drowsiness, etc.) ______________________________

____

Discontinued Date ______________ ❑ Monthly prescription refill

Reason: ❑ Completed ❑ Reaction: *Be sure to add to Allergy Section - Medication.*

Medication Records

Date ____________ Dr. ______________________________ Phone ( ) ____________

Medication ______________________________________ Rx # ____________

Purpose ____

Dosage ________ mg _____ Length *(days)* ________ Other ____________

Time

				Other

Special instructions *(i.e., taken with food, increase water, etc.)* ____________

____

Side effects (i.e., may cause drowsiness, etc.) ____________

____

Discontinued Date ____________ ❑ Monthly prescription refill

Reason: ❑ Completed ❑ Reaction: *Be sure to add to Allergy Section - Medication.*

Date ____________ Dr. ______________________________ Phone ( ) ____________

Medication ______________________________________ Rx # ____________

Purpose ____

Dosage ________ mg _____ Length *(days)* ________ Other ____________

Time

				Other

Special instructions *(i.e., taken with food, increase water, etc.)* ____________

____

Side effects (i.e., may cause drowsiness, etc.) ____________

____

Discontinued Date ____________ ❑ Monthly prescription refill

Reason: ❑ Completed ❑ Reaction: *Be sure to add to Allergy Section - Medication.*

Date ____________ Dr. ______________________________ Phone ( ) ____________

Medication ______________________________________ Rx # ____________

Purpose ____

Dosage ________ mg _____ Length *(days)* ________ Other ____________

Time

				Other

Special instructions *(i.e., taken with food, increase water, etc.)* ____________

____

Side effects (i.e., may cause drowsiness, etc.) ____________

____

Discontinued Date ____________ ❑ Monthly prescription refill

Reason: ❑ Completed ❑ Reaction: *Be sure to add to Allergy Section - Medication.*

Medication Records

Date ____________ Dr. ____________________________ Phone (   ) ____________

Medication ____________________________________ Rx # ____________

Purpose ____

Dosage __________ mg _____ Length *(days)* ____________ Other ____________

Time

				Other

Special instructions *(i.e., taken with food, increase water, etc.)* ____________

____

Side effects (i.e., may cause drowsiness, etc.) ____________

____

Discontinued Date ____________ ❑ Monthly prescription refill

Reason: ❑ Completed ❑ Reaction: *Be sure to add to Allergy Section - Medication.*

Date ____________ Dr. ____________________________ Phone (   ) ____________

Medication ____________________________________ Rx # ____________

Purpose ____

Dosage __________ mg _____ Length *(days)* ____________ Other ____________

Time

				Other

Special instructions *(i.e., taken with food, increase water, etc.)* ____________

____

Side effects (i.e., may cause drowsiness, etc.) ____________

____

Discontinued Date ____________ ❑ Monthly prescription refill

Reason: ❑ Completed ❑ Reaction: *Be sure to add to Allergy Section - Medication.*

Date ____________ Dr. ____________________________ Phone (   ) ____________

Medication ____________________________________ Rx # ____________

Purpose ____

Dosage __________ mg _____ Length *(days)* ____________ Other ____________

Time

				Other

Special instructions *(i.e., taken with food, increase water, etc.)* ____________

____

Side effects (i.e., may cause drowsiness, etc.) ____________

____

Discontinued Date ____________ ❑ Monthly prescription refill

Reason: ❑ Completed ❑ Reaction: *Be sure to add to Allergy Section - Medication.*

Medication Records

Date ______________ Dr. ________________________________ Phone ( ) ______________

Medication ____ Rx # ______________

Purpose ____

Dosage ____________ mg _____ Length *(days)* ______________ Other ______________

Time

				Other

Special instructions *(i.e., taken with food, increase water, etc.)* ______________

____

Side effects (i.e., may cause drowsiness, etc.) ______________________________

____

Discontinued Date ______________________ ❑ Monthly prescription refill

Reason: ❑ Completed ❑ Reaction: *Be sure to add to Allergy Section - Medication.*

Date ______________ Dr. ________________________________ Phone ( ) ______________

Medication ____ Rx # ______________

Purpose ____

Dosage ____________ mg _____ Length *(days)* ______________ Other ______________

Time

				Other

Special instructions *(i.e., taken with food, increase water, etc.)* ______________

____

Side effects (i.e., may cause drowsiness, etc.) ______________________________

____

Discontinued Date ______________________ ❑ Monthly prescription refill

Reason: ❑ Completed ❑ Reaction: *Be sure to add to Allergy Section - Medication.*

Date ______________ Dr. ________________________________ Phone ( ) ______________

Medication ____ Rx # ______________

Purpose ____

Dosage ____________ mg _____ Length *(days)* ______________ Other ______________

Time

				Other

Special instructions *(i.e., taken with food, increase water, etc.)* ______________

____

Side effects (i.e., may cause drowsiness, etc.) ______________________________

____

Discontinued Date ______________________ ❑ Monthly prescription refill

Reason: ❑ Completed ❑ Reaction: *Be sure to add to Allergy Section - Medication.*

Medications

Medication Records

Date ______ Dr. ______ Phone ( ) ______

Medication ______ Rx # ______

Purpose ______

Dosage ______ mg ______ Length *(days)* ______ Other ______

Time

				Other

Special instructions *(i.e., taken with food, increase water, etc.)* ______

Side effects (i.e., may cause drowsiness, etc.) ______

Discontinued Date ______ ❑ Monthly prescription refill

Reason: ❑ Completed ❑ Reaction: *Be sure to add to Allergy Section - Medication.*

Date ______ Dr. ______ Phone ( ) ______

Medication ______ Rx # ______

Purpose ______

Dosage ______ mg ______ Length *(days)* ______ Other ______

Time

				Other

Special instructions *(i.e., taken with food, increase water, etc.)* ______

Side effects (i.e., may cause drowsiness, etc.) ______

Discontinued Date ______ ❑ Monthly prescription refill

Reason: ❑ Completed ❑ Reaction: *Be sure to add to Allergy Section - Medication.*

Date ______ Dr. ______ Phone ( ) ______

Medication ______ Rx # ______

Purpose ______

Dosage ______ mg ______ Length *(days)* ______ Other ______

Time

				Other

Special instructions *(i.e., taken with food, increase water, etc.)* ______

Side effects (i.e., may cause drowsiness, etc.) ______

Discontinued Date ______ ❑ Monthly prescription refill

Reason: ❑ Completed ❑ Reaction: *Be sure to add to Allergy Section - Medication.*

Medication Records

Date ______________ Dr. ________________________________ Phone (   ) ______________

Medication ____ Rx # ______________

Purpose ____

Dosage ____________ mg _____ Length *(days)* ____________ Other ______________

Time

				Other

Special instructions *(i.e., taken with food, increase water, etc.)* ______________

____

Side effects (i.e., may cause drowsiness, etc.) ______________

____

Discontinued Date ______________ ❑ Monthly prescription refill

Reason: ❑ Completed ❑ Reaction: *Be sure to add to Allergy Section - Medication.*

Date ______________ Dr. ________________________________ Phone (   ) ______________

Medication ____ Rx # ______________

Purpose ____

Dosage ____________ mg _____ Length *(days)* ____________ Other ______________

Time

				Other

Special instructions *(i.e., taken with food, increase water, etc.)* ______________

____

Side effects (i.e., may cause drowsiness, etc.) ______________

____

Discontinued Date ______________ ❑ Monthly prescription refill

Reason: ❑ Completed ❑ Reaction: *Be sure to add to Allergy Section - Medication.*

Date ______________ Dr. ________________________________ Phone (   ) ______________

Medication ____ Rx # ______________

Purpose ____

Dosage ____________ mg _____ Length *(days)* ____________ Other ______________

Time

				Other

Special instructions *(i.e., taken with food, increase water, etc.)* ______________

____

Side effects (i.e., may cause drowsiness, etc.) ______________

____

Discontinued Date ______________ ❑ Monthly prescription refill

Reason: ❑ Completed ❑ Reaction: *Be sure to add to Allergy Section - Medication.*

Medication Records

Date ______________ Dr. ________________________________ Phone (   ) ______________

Medication ____ Rx # ______________

Purpose ____

Dosage __________ mg _____ Length *(days)* __________ Other ______________

Time

				Other

Special instructions *(i.e., taken with food, increase water, etc.)* ______________________

____

Side effects (i.e., may cause drowsiness, etc.) ______________________

____

Discontinued Date ______________ ❑ Monthly prescription refill

Reason: ❑ Completed ❑ Reaction: *Be sure to add to Allergy Section - Medication.*

Date ______________ Dr. ________________________________ Phone (   ) ______________

Medication ____ Rx # ______________

Purpose ____

Dosage __________ mg _____ Length *(days)* __________ Other ______________

Time

				Other

Special instructions *(i.e., taken with food, increase water, etc.)* ______________________

____

Side effects (i.e., may cause drowsiness, etc.) ______________________

____

Discontinued Date ______________ ❑ Monthly prescription refill

Reason: ❑ Completed ❑ Reaction: *Be sure to add to Allergy Section - Medication.*

Date ______________ Dr. ________________________________ Phone (   ) ______________

Medication ____ Rx # ______________

Purpose ____

Dosage __________ mg _____ Length *(days)* __________ Other ______________

Time

				Other

Special instructions *(i.e., taken with food, increase water, etc.)* ______________________

____

Side effects (i.e., may cause drowsiness, etc.) ______________________

____

Discontinued Date ______________ ❑ Monthly prescription refill

Reason: ❑ Completed ❑ Reaction: *Be sure to add to Allergy Section - Medication.*

Medication Daily Schedule

Place the time and date in appropriate box.

Medication ______________________ Date started ______________________

Time

				Other

Discontinued Date ________ ❑ Monthly prescription refill Rx # ______________________
Reason: ❑ Completed ❑ Reaction: *Be sure to add to Allergy Section - Medication.*

Medication ______________________ Date started ______________________

Time

				Other

Discontinued Date ________ ❑ Monthly prescription refill Rx # ______________________
Reason: ❑ Completed ❑ Reaction: *Be sure to add to Allergy Section - Medication.*

Medication ______________________ Date started ______________________

Time

				Other

Discontinued Date ________ ❑ Monthly prescription refill Rx # ______________________
Reason: ❑ Completed ❑ Reaction: *Be sure to add to Allergy Section - Medication.*

Medication ______________________ Date started ______________________

Time

				Other

Discontinued Date ________ ❑ Monthly prescription refill Rx # ______________________
Reason: ❑ Completed ❑ Reaction: *Be sure to add to Allergy Section - Medication.*

Medication ______________________ Date started ______________________

Time

				Other

Discontinued Date ________ ❑ Monthly prescription refill Rx # ______________________
Reason: ❑ Completed ❑ Reaction: *Be sure to add to Allergy Section - Medication.*

Medication ______________________ Date started ______________________

Time

				Other

Discontinued Date ________ ❑ Monthly prescription refill Rx # ______________________
Reason: ❑ Completed ❑ Reaction: *Be sure to add to Allergy Section - Medication.*

Medication ______________________ Date started ______________________

Time

				Other

Discontinued Date ________ ❑ Monthly prescription refill Rx # ______________________
Reason: ❑ Completed ❑ Reaction: *Be sure to add to Allergy Section - Medication.*

Medication Daily Schedule

Place the time and date in appropriate box.

Medication ______________________ Date started ______________________

Time

				Other

Discontinued Date __________ ❑ Monthly prescription refill Rx # ______________________

Reason: ❑ Completed ❑ Reaction: *Be sure to add to Allergy Section - Medication.*

Medication ______________________ Date started ______________________

Time

				Other

Discontinued Date __________ ❑ Monthly prescription refill Rx # ______________________

Reason: ❑ Completed ❑ Reaction: *Be sure to add to Allergy Section - Medication.*

Medication ______________________ Date started ______________________

Time

				Other

Discontinued Date __________ ❑ Monthly prescription refill Rx # ______________________

Reason: ❑ Completed ❑ Reaction: *Be sure to add to Allergy Section - Medication.*

Medication ______________________ Date started ______________________

Time

				Other

Discontinued Date __________ ❑ Monthly prescription refill Rx # ______________________

Reason: ❑ Completed ❑ Reaction: *Be sure to add to Allergy Section - Medication.*

Medication ______________________ Date started ______________________

Time

				Other

Discontinued Date __________ ❑ Monthly prescription refill Rx # ______________________

Reason: ❑ Completed ❑ Reaction: *Be sure to add to Allergy Section - Medication.*

Medication ______________________ Date started ______________________

Time

				Other

Discontinued Date __________ ❑ Monthly prescription refill Rx # ______________________

Reason: ❑ Completed ❑ Reaction: *Be sure to add to Allergy Section - Medication.*

Medication ______________________ Date started ______________________

Time

				Other

Discontinued Date __________ ❑ Monthly prescription refill Rx # ______________________

Reason: ❑ Completed ❑ Reaction: *Be sure to add to Allergy Section - Medication.*

Medication Daily Schedule

Place the time and date in appropriate box.

Medication ______________________ Date started ______________________

Time

				Other

Discontinued Date __________ ❑ Monthly prescription refill Rx # ______________

Reason: ❑ Completed ❑ Reaction: *Be sure to add to Allergy Section - Medication.*

Medication ______________________ Date started ______________________

Time

				Other

Discontinued Date __________ ❑ Monthly prescription refill Rx # ______________

Reason: ❑ Completed ❑ Reaction: *Be sure to add to Allergy Section - Medication.*

Medication ______________________ Date started ______________________

Time

				Other

Discontinued Date __________ ❑ Monthly prescription refill Rx # ______________

Reason: ❑ Completed ❑ Reaction: *Be sure to add to Allergy Section - Medication.*

Medication ______________________ Date started ______________________

Time

				Other

Discontinued Date __________ ❑ Monthly prescription refill Rx # ______________

Reason: ❑ Completed ❑ Reaction: *Be sure to add to Allergy Section - Medication.*

Medication ______________________ Date started ______________________

Time

				Other

Discontinued Date __________ ❑ Monthly prescription refill Rx # ______________

Reason: ❑ Completed ❑ Reaction: *Be sure to add to Allergy Section - Medication.*

Medication ______________________ Date started ______________________

Time

				Other

Discontinued Date __________ ❑ Monthly prescription refill Rx # ______________

Reason: ❑ Completed ❑ Reaction: *Be sure to add to Allergy Section - Medication.*

Medication ______________________ Date started ______________________

Time

				Other

Discontinued Date __________ ❑ Monthly prescription refill Rx # ______________

Reason: ❑ Completed ❑ Reaction: *Be sure to add to Allergy Section - Medication.*

Medication Daily Schedule

Place the time and date in appropriate box.

Medication ________________ Date started ________________

Time

				Other

Discontinued Date ________ ❑ Monthly prescription refill Rx # ________________
Reason: ❑ Completed ❑ Reaction: *Be sure to add to Allergy Section - Medication.*

Medication ________________ Date started ________________

Time

				Other

Discontinued Date ________ ❑ Monthly prescription refill Rx # ________________
Reason: ❑ Completed ❑ Reaction: *Be sure to add to Allergy Section - Medication.*

Medication ________________ Date started ________________

Time

				Other

Discontinued Date ________ ❑ Monthly prescription refill Rx # ________________
Reason: ❑ Completed ❑ Reaction: *Be sure to add to Allergy Section - Medication.*

Medication ________________ Date started ________________

Time

				Other

Discontinued Date ________ ❑ Monthly prescription refill Rx # ________________
Reason: ❑ Completed ❑ Reaction: *Be sure to add to Allergy Section - Medication.*

Medication ________________ Date started ________________

Time

				Other

Discontinued Date ________ ❑ Monthly prescription refill Rx # ________________
Reason: ❑ Completed ❑ Reaction: *Be sure to add to Allergy Section - Medication.*

Medication ________________ Date started ________________

Time

				Other

Discontinued Date ________ ❑ Monthly prescription refill Rx # ________________
Reason: ❑ Completed ❑ Reaction: *Be sure to add to Allergy Section - Medication.*

Medication ________________ Date started ________________

Time

				Other

Discontinued Date ________ ❑ Monthly prescription refill Rx # ________________
Reason: ❑ Completed ❑ Reaction: *Be sure to add to Allergy Section - Medication.*

Medication Daily Schedule

Place the time and date in appropriate box.

Medication ______________________ Date started ______________________

Time

				Other

Discontinued Date __________ ❑ Monthly prescription refill Rx # ______________________
Reason: ❑ Completed ❑ Reaction: *Be sure to add to Allergy Section - Medication.*

Medication ______________________ Date started ______________________

Time

				Other

Discontinued Date __________ ❑ Monthly prescription refill Rx # ______________________
Reason: ❑ Completed ❑ Reaction: *Be sure to add to Allergy Section - Medication.*

Medication ______________________ Date started ______________________

Time

				Other

Discontinued Date __________ ❑ Monthly prescription refill Rx # ______________________
Reason: ❑ Completed ❑ Reaction: *Be sure to add to Allergy Section - Medication.*

Medication ______________________ Date started ______________________

Time

				Other

Discontinued Date __________ ❑ Monthly prescription refill Rx # ______________________
Reason: ❑ Completed ❑ Reaction: *Be sure to add to Allergy Section - Medication.*

Medication ______________________ Date started ______________________

Time

				Other

Discontinued Date __________ ❑ Monthly prescription refill Rx # ______________________
Reason: ❑ Completed ❑ Reaction: *Be sure to add to Allergy Section - Medication.*

Medication ______________________ Date started ______________________

Time

				Other

Discontinued Date __________ ❑ Monthly prescription refill Rx # ______________________
Reason: ❑ Completed ❑ Reaction: *Be sure to add to Allergy Section - Medication.*

Medication ______________________ Date started ______________________

Time

				Other

Discontinued Date __________ ❑ Monthly prescription refill Rx # ______________________
Reason: ❑ Completed ❑ Reaction: *Be sure to add to Allergy Section - Medication.*

Medication Daily Schedule

Place the time and date in appropriate box.

Medication ______________________ Date started ______________________

Time

				Other

Discontinued Date __________ ❑ Monthly prescription refill Rx #______________________
Reason: ❑ Completed ❑ Reaction: *Be sure to add to Allergy Section - Medication.*

Medication ______________________ Date started ______________________

Time

				Other

Discontinued Date __________ ❑ Monthly prescription refill Rx #______________________
Reason: ❑ Completed ❑ Reaction: *Be sure to add to Allergy Section - Medication.*

Medication ______________________ Date started ______________________

Time

				Other

Discontinued Date __________ ❑ Monthly prescription refill Rx #______________________
Reason: ❑ Completed ❑ Reaction: *Be sure to add to Allergy Section - Medication.*

Medication ______________________ Date started ______________________

Time

				Other

Discontinued Date __________ ❑ Monthly prescription refill Rx #______________________
Reason: ❑ Completed ❑ Reaction: *Be sure to add to Allergy Section - Medication.*

Medication ______________________ Date started ______________________

Time

				Other

Discontinued Date __________ ❑ Monthly prescription refill Rx #______________________
Reason: ❑ Completed ❑ Reaction: *Be sure to add to Allergy Section - Medication.*

Medication ______________________ Date started ______________________

Time

				Other

Discontinued Date __________ ❑ Monthly prescription refill Rx #______________________
Reason: ❑ Completed ❑ Reaction: *Be sure to add to Allergy Section - Medication.*

Medication ______________________ Date started ______________________

Time

				Other

Discontinued Date __________ ❑ Monthly prescription refill Rx #______________________
Reason: ❑ Completed ❑ Reaction: *Be sure to add to Allergy Section - Medication.*

ALLERGIES – MEDICATION * FOOD * OTHER LOG AND RECORD

Log

Maintain a log of your allergies for easy access.

Records

Be sure to write down any allergic reactions, and what medication or treatment is necessary to resolve this problem. This is extremely vital for any medical professional who is assisting you.

Notes

Allergies

Allergy Log

Maintain a log for easy recall and review.

❑ **MEDICATION** ❑ **FOOD** ❑ **OTHER**

Best to use a separate page for each category.

Date	Name	Reaction

Allergies

Allergy Log

Maintain a log for easy recall and review.

❏ **MEDICATION** ❏ **FOOD** ❏ **OTHER**

Best to use a separate page for each category.

Date	Name	Reaction

Allergies

Allergy Log

Maintain a log for easy recall and review.

❑ **MEDICATION** ❑ **FOOD** ❑ **OTHER**

Best to use a separate page for each category.

Date	Name	Reaction

Allergies

Allergy Log

Maintain a log for easy recall and review.

❑ **MEDICATION** ❑ **FOOD** ❑ **OTHER**

Best to use a separate page for each category.

Date	Name	Reaction

Allergies

Allergy Records

❑ **MEDICATION** ❑ **FOOD** ❑ **OTHER**

Best to use a separate page for each category.

Date ______________________ Type ______________________

Reaction ____

Counteraction / Dosage __________________________________

____

Dr. ______________________ Medical Facility ______________

Date ______________________ Type ______________________

Reaction ____

Counteraction / Dosage __________________________________

____

Dr. ______________________ Medical Facility ______________

Date ______________________ Type ______________________

Reaction ____

Counteraction / Dosage __________________________________

____

Dr. ______________________ Medical Facility ______________

Date ______________________ Type ______________________

Reaction ____

Counteraction / Dosage __________________________________

____

Dr. ______________________ Medical Facility ______________

Date ______________________ Type ______________________

Reaction ____

Counteraction / Dosage __________________________________

____

Dr. ______________________ Medical Facility ______________

Allergy Records

❑ **MEDICATION** ❑ **FOOD** ❑ **OTHER**

Best to use a separate page for each category.

Date ______________________ Type ______________________

Reaction ______________________

Counteraction / Dosage ______________________

____

Dr. ______________________ Medical Facility ______________________

Date ______________________ Type ______________________

Reaction ______________________

Counteraction / Dosage ______________________

____

Dr. ______________________ Medical Facility ______________________

Date ______________________ Type ______________________

Reaction ______________________

Counteraction / Dosage ______________________

____

Dr. ______________________ Medical Facility ______________________

Date ______________________ Type ______________________

Reaction ______________________

Counteraction / Dosage ______________________

____

Dr. ______________________ Medical Facility ______________________

Date ______________________ Type ______________________

Reaction ______________________

Counteraction / Dosage ______________________

____

Dr. ______________________ Medical Facility ______________________

Allergy Records

❑ **MEDICATION** ❑ **FOOD** ❑ **OTHER**

Best to use a separate page for each category.

Date ______________________ Type ______________________

Reaction ______________________

Counteraction / Dosage ______________________

____

Dr. ______________________ Medical Facility ______________________

Date ______________________ Type ______________________

Reaction ______________________

Counteraction / Dosage ______________________

____

Dr. ______________________ Medical Facility ______________________

Date ______________________ Type ______________________

Reaction ______________________

Counteraction / Dosage ______________________

____

Dr. ______________________ Medical Facility ______________________

Date ______________________ Type ______________________

Reaction ______________________

Counteraction / Dosage ______________________

____

Dr. ______________________ Medical Facility ______________________

Date ______________________ Type ______________________

Reaction ______________________

Counteraction / Dosage ______________________

____

Dr. ______________________ Medical Facility ______________________

Allergy Records

❑ **MEDICATION** ❑ **FOOD** ❑ **OTHER**

Best to use a separate page for each category.

Date ______________________ Type ______________________

Reaction ______________________

Counteraction / Dosage ______________________

____

Dr. ______________________ Medical Facility ______________________

Date ______________________ Type ______________________

Reaction ______________________

Counteraction / Dosage ______________________

____

Dr. ______________________ Medical Facility ______________________

Date ______________________ Type ______________________

Reaction ______________________

Counteraction / Dosage ______________________

____

Dr. ______________________ Medical Facility ______________________

Date ______________________ Type ______________________

Reaction ______________________

Counteraction / Dosage ______________________

____

Dr. ______________________ Medical Facility ______________________

Date ______________________ Type ______________________

Reaction ______________________

Counteraction / Dosage ______________________

____

Dr. ______________________ Medical Facility ______________________

Hospitalizations * Surgeries * Procedures Log and Records

Log

Maintain a log for easy recall and review.

Records

It is beneficial that you, the physician, or the dentist, summarize the procedure, complications, and any notes in this area.

Ask for a copy of the Doctor's surgical or procedure notes for your file or binder.

Notes

Hospitalizations * Surgeries * Procedures Log

Place a (✓) in the appropriate category.

DATE	TYPE	HOSPITALIZATION	SURGERY	PROCEDURE	COMMENTS

Hospitalizations * Surgeries * Procedures Log

Place a (✓) in the appropriate category.

DATE	TYPE	HOSPITALIZATION	SURGERY	PROCEDURE	COMMENTS

Hospitalizations * Surgeries * Procedures Records

❑ **HOSPITALIZATION** ❑ **SURGERY** ❑ **PROCEDURE**

Best to use a separate page for each category.

Date ____________________ Dr. ____________________

Medical Facility ____________________

City ____________________ State ____________________

Phone (   ) ____________________ Other ____________________

Temperature ____________________ Blood pressure ____________________

Pulse ____________________ Glucose ____________________

Other ____________________

Blood Test ____________________

Anesthesia ____________________ Dr. ____________________

Reaction: ❑ No ❑ Yes ____________________

____

____

Counteraction ____________________

____

____

Procedure ____________________

____

____

Summary ____________________

____

____

Complications ____________________

____

Length of Stay ____________________

____

❑ *See hospital discharge and care instructions.*

Add a separate page if you need to write more detail.

Hospitalizations * Surgeries * Procedures

Hospitalizations * Surgeries * Procedures Records

❑ **HOSPITALIZATION** ❑ **SURGERY** ❑ **PROCEDURE**

Best to use a separate page for each category.

Date ____________ Dr. ____________

Medical Facility ____________

City ____________ State ____________

Phone (   ) ____________ Other ____________

Temperature ____________ Blood pressure ____________

Pulse ____________ Glucose ____________

Other ____________

Blood Test ____________

Anesthesia ____________ Dr. ____________

Reaction: ❑ No ❑ Yes ____________

Counteraction ____________

Procedure ____________

Summary ____________

Complications ____________

Length of Stay ____________

❑ *See hospital discharge and care instructions.*

Add a separate page if you need to write more detail.

Hospitalizations * Surgeries * Procedures Records

❑ **HOSPITALIZATION** ❑ **SURGERY** ❑ **PROCEDURE**

Best to use a separate page for each category.

Date ____________________ Dr. ____

Medical Facility ____

City ________________________________ State ______________________________

Phone (______) ____________________ Other ______________________________

Temperature _________________________ Blood pressure ____________________

Pulse ______________________________ Glucose ___________________________

Other ____

Blood Test ____

Anesthesia __________________________ Dr. _______________________________

Reaction: ❑ No ❑ Yes ____

____

____

Counteraction ____

____

____

Procedure ____

____

____

Summary ____

____

____

Complications ____

____

Length of Stay ____

____

❑ *See hospital discharge and care instructions.*

Add a separate page if you need to write more detail.

Hospitalizations * Surgeries * Procedures Records

❑ **HOSPITALIZATION** ❑ **SURGERY** ❑ **PROCEDURE**

Best to use a separate page for each category.

Date ____________ Dr. ____________

Medical Facility ____________

City ____________ State ____________

Phone (   ) ____________ Other ____________

Temperature ____________ Blood pressure ____________

Pulse ____________ Glucose ____________

Other ____________

Blood Test ____________

Anesthesia ____________ Dr. ____________

Reaction: ❑ No ❑ Yes ____________

____

____

Counteraction ____________

____

____

Procedure ____________

____

____

Summary ____________

____

____

Complications ____________

____

Length of Stay ____________

____

❑ *See hospital discharge and care instructions.*

Add a separate page if you need to write more detail.

Hospitalizations * Surgeries * Procedures Records

❑ **HOSPITALIZATION** ❑ **SURGERY** ❑ **PROCEDURE**

Best to use a separate page for each category.

Date ____________ Dr. ____________

Medical Facility ____________

City ____________ State ____________

Phone (   ) ____________ Other ____________

Temperature ____________ Blood pressure ____________

Pulse ____________ Glucose ____________

Other ____________

Blood Test ____________

Anesthesia ____________ Dr. ____________

Reaction: ❑ No ❑ Yes ____________

Counteraction ____________

Procedure ____________

Summary ____________

Complications ____________

Length of Stay ____________

❑ *See hospital discharge and care instructions.*

Add a separate page if you need to write more detail.

Hospitalizations * Surgeries * Procedures Records

❑ **HOSPITALIZATION** ❑ **SURGERY** ❑ **PROCEDURE**

Best to use a separate page for each category.

Date ________________ Dr. ________________________________

Medical Facility ________________________________

City ________________________ State ________________________

Phone (   ) ____________________ Other ________________________

Temperature ____________________ Blood pressure ____________________

Pulse ________________________ Glucose ________________________

Other ________________________________

Blood Test ________________________________

Anesthesia ____________________ Dr. ________________________

Reaction: ❑ No ❑ Yes ________________________________

____

____

Counteraction ________________________________

____

____

Procedure ________________________________

____

____

Summary ________________________________

____

____

Complications ________________________________

____

Length of Stay ________________________________

____

❑ *See hospital discharge and care instructions.*

Add a separate page if you need to write more detail.

Hospitalizations * Surgeries * Procedures Records

❑ **HOSPITALIZATION** ❑ **SURGERY** ❑ **PROCEDURE**

Best to use a separate page for each category.

Date ____________________ Dr. ____

Medical Facility ____

City ______________________________ State ______________________________

Phone (______) ______________________ Other ______________________________

Temperature ______________________ Blood pressure ______________________

Pulse ______________________________ Glucose ______________________________

Other ____

Blood Test ____

Anesthesia ______________________________ Dr. ______________________________

Reaction: ❑ No ❑ Yes ____

____

____

Counteraction ____

____

____

Procedure ____

____

____

Summary ____

____

____

Complications ____

____

Length of Stay ____

____

❑ *See hospital discharge and care instructions.*

Add a separate page if you need to write more detail.

Hospitalizations * Surgeries * Procedures Records

❑ **HOSPITALIZATION** ❑ **SURGERY** ❑ **PROCEDURE**

Best to use a separate page for each category.

Date ____________ Dr. ____________

Medical Facility ____________

City ____________ State ____________

Phone (   ) ____________ Other ____________

Temperature ____________ Blood pressure ____________

Pulse ____________ Glucose ____________

Other ____________

Blood Test ____________

Anesthesia ____________ Dr. ____________

Reaction: ❑ No ❑ Yes ____________

____

____

Counteraction ____________

____

____

Procedure ____________

____

____

Summary ____________

____

____

Complications ____________

____

Length of Stay ____________

____

❑ *See hospital discharge and care instructions.*

Add a separate page if you need to write more detail.

Hospitalizations * Surgeries * Procedures Records

❑ **HOSPITALIZATION** ❑ **SURGERY** ❑ **PROCEDURE**

Best to use a separate page for each category.

Date ____________________ Dr. ____________________

Medical Facility ____________________

City ____________________ State ____________________

Phone (   ) ____________________ Other ____________________

Temperature ____________________ Blood pressure ____________________

Pulse ____________________ Glucose ____________________

Other ____________________

Blood Test ____________________

Anesthesia ____________________ Dr. ____________________

Reaction: ❑ No ❑ Yes ____________________

____

____

Counteraction ____________________

____

____

Procedure ____________________

____

____

Summary ____________________

____

____

Complications ____________________

____

Length of Stay ____________________

____

❑ *See hospital discharge and care instructions.*

Add a separate page if you need to write more detail.

Hospitalizations * Surgeries * Procedures Records

❑ **HOSPITALIZATION** ❑ **SURGERY** ❑ **PROCEDURE**

Best to use a separate page for each category.

Date ____________________ Dr. ____________________

Medical Facility ____________________

City ____________________ State ____________________

Phone (   ) ____________________ Other ____________________

Temperature ____________________ Blood pressure ____________________

Pulse ____________________ Glucose ____________________

Other ____________________

Blood Test ____________________

Anesthesia ____________________ Dr. ____________________

Reaction: ❑ No ❑ Yes ____________________

____

____

Counteraction ____________________

____

____

Procedure ____________________

____

____

Summary ____________________

____

____

Complications ____________________

____

Length of Stay ____________________

____

❑ *See hospital discharge and care instructions.*

Add a separate page if you need to write more detail.

Hospitalizations * Surgeries * Procedures Records

❑ **HOSPITALIZATION** ❑ **SURGERY** ❑ **PROCEDURE**

Best to use a separate page for each category.

Date ____________________ Dr. ____________________

Medical Facility ____________________

City ____________________ State ____________________

Phone (______) ____________________ Other ____________________

Temperature ____________________ Blood pressure ____________________

Pulse ____________________ Glucose ____________________

Other ____________________

Blood Test ____________________

Anesthesia ____________________ Dr. ____________________

Reaction: ❑ No ❑ Yes ____________________

____

____

Counteraction ____________________

____

____

Procedure ____________________

____

____

Summary ____________________

____

____

Complications ____________________

____

Length of Stay ____________________

____

❑ *See hospital discharge and care instructions.*

Add a separate page if you need to write more detail.

Hospitalizations * Surgeries * Procedures Records

❑ **HOSPITALIZATION** ❑ **SURGERY** ❑ **PROCEDURE**

Best to use a separate page for each category.

Date ____________________ Dr. ____________________

Medical Facility ____________________

City ____________________ State ____________________

Phone (   ) ____________________ Other ____________________

Temperature ____________________ Blood pressure ____________________

Pulse ____________________ Glucose ____________________

Other ____________________

Blood Test ____________________

Anesthesia ____________________ Dr. ____________________

Reaction: ❑ No ❑ Yes ____________________

____

____

Counteraction ____________________

____

____

Procedure ____________________

____

____

Summary ____________________

____

____

Complications ____________________

____

Length of Stay ____________________

____

❑ *See hospital discharge and care instructions.*

Add a separate page if you need to write more detail.

Hospitalizations * Surgeries * Procedures Records

❑ **HOSPITALIZATION** ❑ **SURGERY** ❑ **PROCEDURE**

Best to use a separate page for each category.

Date ____________________ Dr. ____

Medical Facility ____

City ____________________ State ____________________

Phone (   ) ____________________ Other ____________________

Temperature ____________________ Blood pressure ____________________

Pulse ____________________ Glucose ____________________

Other ____

Blood Test ____

Anesthesia ____________________ Dr. ____________________

Reaction: ❑ No ❑ Yes ____

____

____

Counteraction ____

____

____

Procedure ____

____

____

Summary ____

____

____

Complications ____

____

Length of Stay ____

____

❑ *See hospital discharge and care instructions.*

Add a separate page if you need to write more detail.

Hospitalizations * Surgeries * Procedures Records

❑ **HOSPITALIZATION** ❑ **SURGERY** ❑ **PROCEDURE**

Best to use a separate page for each category.

Date ________________ Dr. ________________________________

Medical Facility ________________________________

City ________________________ State ________________________

Phone (   ) ________________________ Other ________________________

Temperature ________________________ Blood pressure ________________________

Pulse ________________________ Glucose ________________________

Other ________________________________

Blood Test ________________________________

Anesthesia ________________________ Dr. ________________________

Reaction: ❑ No ❑ Yes ________________________________

____

____

Counteraction ________________________________

____

____

Procedure ________________________________

____

____

Summary ________________________________

____

____

Complications ________________________________

____

Length of Stay ________________________________

____

❑ *See hospital discharge and care instructions.*

Add a separate page if you need to write more detail.

Hospitalizations * Surgeries * Procedures Records

❑ **HOSPITALIZATION** ❑ **SURGERY** ❑ **PROCEDURE**

Best to use a separate page for each category.

Date ____________ Dr. ____________

Medical Facility ____________

City ____________ State ____________

Phone (   ) ____________ Other ____________

Temperature ____________ Blood pressure ____________

Pulse ____________ Glucose ____________

Other ____________

Blood Test ____________

Anesthesia ____________ Dr. ____________

Reaction: ❑ No ❑ Yes ____________

Counteraction ____________

Procedure ____________

Summary ____________

Complications ____________

Length of Stay ____________

❑ *See hospital discharge and care instructions.*

Add a separate page if you need to write more detail.

Hospitalizations * Surgeries * Procedures Records

❑ **HOSPITALIZATION** ❑ **SURGERY** ❑ **PROCEDURE**

Best to use a separate page for each category.

Date ____________ Dr. ____________

Medical Facility ____________

City ____________ State ____________

Phone (   ) ____________ Other ____________

Temperature ____________ Blood pressure ____________

Pulse ____________ Glucose ____________

Other ____________

Blood Test ____________

Anesthesia ____________ Dr. ____________

Reaction: ❑ No ❑ Yes ____________

Counteraction ____________

Procedure ____________

Summary ____________

Complications ____________

Length of Stay ____________

❑ *See hospital discharge and care instructions.*

Add a separate page if you need to write more detail.

Hospitalizations * Surgeries * Procedures Records

❑ **HOSPITALIZATION** ❑ **SURGERY** ❑ **PROCEDURE**

Best to use a separate page for each category.

Date ____________________ Dr. ______________________________

Medical Facility ______________________________

City ____________________ State ____________________

Phone (   ) ____________________ Other ____________________

Temperature ____________________ Blood pressure ____________________

Pulse ____________________ Glucose ____________________

Other ______________________________

Blood Test ______________________________

Anesthesia ____________________ Dr. ____________________

Reaction: ❑ No ❑ Yes ______________________________

____

____

Counteraction ______________________________

____

____

Procedure ______________________________

____

____

Summary ______________________________

____

____

Complications ______________________________

____

Length of Stay ______________________________

____

❑ *See hospital discharge and care instructions.*

Add a separate page if you need to write more detail.

Hospitalizations * Surgeries * Procedures Records

❑ **HOSPITALIZATION** ❑ **SURGERY** ❑ **PROCEDURE**

Best to use a separate page for each category.

Date ____________ Dr. ____________

Medical Facility ____________

City ____________ State ____________

Phone (   ) ____________ Other ____________

Temperature ____________ Blood pressure ____________

Pulse ____________ Glucose ____________

Other ____________

Blood Test ____________

Anesthesia ____________ Dr. ____________

Reaction: ❑ No ❑ Yes ____________

Counteraction ____________

Procedure ____________

Summary ____________

Complications ____________

Length of Stay ____________

❑ *See hospital discharge and care instructions.*

Add a separate page if you need to write more detail.

Hospitalizations * Surgeries * Procedures Records

❑ **HOSPITALIZATION** ❑ **SURGERY** ❑ **PROCEDURE**

Best to use a separate page for each category.

Date ____________ Dr. ____________

Medical Facility ____________

City ____________ State ____________

Phone (   ) ____________ Other ____________

Temperature ____________ Blood pressure ____________

Pulse ____________ Glucose ____________

Other ____________

Blood Test ____________

Anesthesia ____________ Dr. ____________

Reaction: ❑ No ❑ Yes ____________

Counteraction ____________

Procedure ____________

Summary ____________

Complications ____________

Length of Stay ____________

❑ *See hospital discharge and care instructions.*

Add a separate page if you need to write more detail.

Hospitalizations * Surgeries * Procedures Records

❑ **HOSPITALIZATION** ❑ **SURGERY** ❑ **PROCEDURE**

Best to use a separate page for each category.

Date ____________ Dr. ____________

Medical Facility ____________

City ____________ State ____________

Phone (   ) ____________ Other ____________

Temperature ____________ Blood pressure ____________

Pulse ____________ Glucose ____________

Other ____________

Blood Test ____________

Anesthesia ____________ Dr. ____________

Reaction: ❑ No ❑ Yes ____________

Counteraction ____________

Procedure ____________

Summary ____________

Complications ____________

Length of Stay ____________

❑ *See hospital discharge and care instructions.*

Add a separate page if you need to write more detail.

Hospitalizations * Surgeries * Procedures Records

❑ **HOSPITALIZATION** ❑ **SURGERY** ❑ **PROCEDURE**

Best to use a separate page for each category.

Date ____________________ Dr. ____________________

Medical Facility ____________________

City ____________________ State ____________________

Phone (   ) ____________________ Other ____________________

Temperature ____________________ Blood pressure ____________________

Pulse ____________________ Glucose ____________________

Other ____________________

Blood Test ____________________

Anesthesia ____________________ Dr. ____________________

Reaction: ❑ No ❑ Yes ____________________

____

____

Counteraction ____________________

____

____

Procedure ____________________

____

____

Summary ____________________

____

____

Complications ____________________

____

Length of Stay ____________________

____

❑ *See hospital discharge and care instructions.*

Add a separate page if you need to write more detail.

Hospitalizations * Surgeries * Procedures Records

❑ **HOSPITALIZATION** ❑ **SURGERY** ❑ **PROCEDURE**

Best to use a separate page for each category.

Date ______________ Dr. ______________

Medical Facility ______________

City ______________ State ______________

Phone (   ) ______________ Other ______________

Temperature ______________ Blood pressure ______________

Pulse ______________ Glucose ______________

Other ______________

Blood Test ______________

Anesthesia ______________ Dr. ______________

Reaction: ❑ No ❑ Yes ______________

____

____

Counteraction ______________

____

____

Procedure ______________

____

____

Summary ______________

____

____

Complications ______________

____

Length of Stay ______________

____

❑ *See hospital discharge and care instructions.*

Add a separate page if you need to write more detail.

Hospitalizations * Surgeries * Procedures Records

❑ **HOSPITALIZATION** ❑ **SURGERY** ❑ **PROCEDURE**

Best to use a separate page for each category.

Date ____________ Dr. ____________

Medical Facility ____________

City ____________ State ____________

Phone (   ) ____________ Other ____________

Temperature ____________ Blood pressure ____________

Pulse ____________ Glucose ____________

Other ____________

Blood Test ____________

Anesthesia ____________ Dr. ____________

Reaction: ❑ No ❑ Yes ____________

____

____

Counteraction ____________

____

____

Procedure ____________

____

____

Summary ____________

____

____

Complications ____________

____

Length of Stay ____________

____

❑ *See hospital discharge and care instructions.*

Add a separate page if you need to write more detail.

Hospitalizations * Surgeries * Procedures Records

❑ **HOSPITALIZATION** ❑ **SURGERY** ❑ **PROCEDURE**

Best to use a separate page for each category.

Date ____________ Dr. ____________

Medical Facility ____________

City ____________ State ____________

Phone (   ) ____________ Other ____________

Temperature ____________ Blood pressure ____________

Pulse ____________ Glucose ____________

Other ____________

Blood Test ____________

Anesthesia ____________ Dr. ____________

Reaction: ❑ No ❑ Yes ____________

Counteraction ____________

Procedure ____________

Summary ____________

Complications ____________

Length of Stay ____________

❑ *See hospital discharge and care instructions.*

Add a separate page if you need to write more detail.

Hospitalizations * Surgeries * Procedures Records

❑ **HOSPITALIZATION** ❑ **SURGERY** ❑ **PROCEDURE**

Best to use a separate page for each category.

Date ____________________ Dr. ______________________________

Medical Facility ______________________________

City ______________________________ State ______________________________

Phone (______) ______________________ Other ______________________________

Temperature ______________________ Blood pressure ______________________

Pulse ______________________________ Glucose ______________________________

Other ______________________________

Blood Test ______________________________

Anesthesia ______________________________ Dr. ______________________________

Reaction: ❑ No ❑ Yes ______________________________

____

____

Counteraction ______________________________

____

____

Procedure ______________________________

____

____

Summary ______________________________

____

____

Complications ______________________________

____

Length of Stay ______________________________

____

❑ *See hospital discharge and care instructions.*

Add a separate page if you need to write more detail.

Hospitalizations * Surgeries * Procedures Records

❑ **HOSPITALIZATION** ❑ **SURGERY** ❑ **PROCEDURE**

Best to use a separate page for each category.

Date ______________ Dr. ______________

Medical Facility ______________

City ______________ State ______________

Phone (   ) ______________ Other ______________

Temperature ______________ Blood pressure ______________

Pulse ______________ Glucose ______________

Other ______________

Blood Test ______________

Anesthesia ______________ Dr. ______________

Reaction: ❑ No ❑ Yes ______________

____

____

Counteraction ______________

____

____

Procedure ______________

____

____

Summary ______________

____

____

Complications ______________

____

Length of Stay ______________

____

❑ *See hospital discharge and care instructions.*

Add a separate page if you need to write more detail.

Hospitalizations * Surgeries * Procedures

Hospitalizations * Surgeries * Procedures Records

❑ **HOSPITALIZATION** ❑ **SURGERY** ❑ **PROCEDURE**

Best to use a separate page for each category.

Date ____________ Dr. ____________

Medical Facility ____________

City ____________ State ____________

Phone (   ) ____________ Other ____________

Temperature ____________ Blood pressure ____________

Pulse ____________ Glucose ____________

Other ____________

Blood Test ____________

Anesthesia ____________ Dr. ____________

Reaction: ❑ No ❑ Yes ____________

Counteraction ____________

Procedure ____________

Summary ____________

Complications ____________

Length of Stay ____________

❑ *See hospital discharge and care instructions.*

Add a separate page if you need to write more detail.

Hospitalizations * Surgeries * Procedures Records

❑ **HOSPITALIZATION** ❑ **SURGERY** ❑ **PROCEDURE**

Best to use a separate page for each category.

Date ____________ Dr. ____________

Medical Facility ____________

City ____________ State ____________

Phone (   ) ____________ Other ____________

Temperature ____________ Blood pressure ____________

Pulse ____________ Glucose ____________

Other ____________

Blood Test ____________

Anesthesia ____________ Dr. ____________

Reaction: ❑ No ❑ Yes ____________

____

____

Counteraction ____________

____

____

Procedure ____________

____

____

Summary ____________

____

____

Complications ____________

____

Length of Stay ____________

____

❑ *See hospital discharge and care instructions.*

Add a separate page if you need to write more detail.

Hospitalizations * Surgeries * Procedures Records

❑ **HOSPITALIZATION** ❑ **SURGERY** ❑ **PROCEDURE**

Best to use a separate page for each category.

Date ____________________ Dr. ____________________

Medical Facility ____________________

City ____________________ State ____________________

Phone (   ) ____________________ Other ____________________

Temperature ____________________ Blood pressure ____________________

Pulse ____________________ Glucose ____________________

Other ____________________

Blood Test ____________________

Anesthesia ____________________ Dr. ____________________

Reaction: ❑ No ❑ Yes ____________________

____

____

Counteraction ____________________

____

____

Procedure ____________________

____

____

Summary ____________________

____

____

Complications ____________________

____

Length of Stay ____________________

____

❑ *See hospital discharge and care instructions.*

Add a separate page if you need to write more detail.

Hospitalizations * Surgeries * Procedures Records

❑ **HOSPITALIZATION** ❑ **SURGERY** ❑ **PROCEDURE**

Best to use a separate page for each category.

Date ____________ Dr. ____________

Medical Facility ____________

City ____________ State ____________

Phone (   ) ____________ Other ____________

Temperature ____________ Blood pressure ____________

Pulse ____________ Glucose ____________

Other ____________

Blood Test ____________

Anesthesia ____________ Dr. ____________

Reaction: ❑ No ❑ Yes ____________

____

____

Counteraction ____________

____

____

Procedure ____________

____

____

Summary ____________

____

____

Complications ____________

____

Length of Stay ____________

____

❑ *See hospital discharge and care instructions.*

Add a separate page if you need to write more detail.

Hospitalizations * Surgeries * Procedures Records

❑ **HOSPITALIZATION** ❑ **SURGERY** ❑ **PROCEDURE**

Best to use a separate page for each category.

Date ____________________ Dr. ____________________

Medical Facility ____________________

City ____________________ State ____________________

Phone (   ) ____________________ Other ____________________

Temperature ____________________ Blood pressure ____________________

Pulse ____________________ Glucose ____________________

Other ____________________

Blood Test ____________________

Anesthesia ____________________ Dr. ____________________

Reaction: ❑ No ❑ Yes ____________________

____

____

Counteraction ____________________

____

____

Procedure ____________________

____

____

Summary ____________________

____

____

Complications ____________________

____

Length of Stay ____________________

____

❑ *See hospital discharge and care instructions.*

Add a separate page if you need to write more detail.

Hospitalizations * Surgeries * Procedures Records

❑ **HOSPITALIZATION** ❑ **SURGERY** ❑ **PROCEDURE**

Best to use a separate page for each category.

Date ____________ Dr. ____________

Medical Facility ____________

City ____________ State ____________

Phone (   ) ____________ Other ____________

Temperature ____________ Blood pressure ____________

Pulse ____________ Glucose ____________

Other ____________

Blood Test ____________

Anesthesia ____________ Dr. ____________

Reaction: ❑ No ❑ Yes ____________

Counteraction ____________

Procedure ____________

Summary ____________

Complications ____________

Length of Stay ____________

❑ *See hospital discharge and care instructions.*

Add a separate page if you need to write more detail.

Hospitalizations * Surgeries * Procedures Records

❑ **HOSPITALIZATION** ❑ **SURGERY** ❑ **PROCEDURE**

Best to use a separate page for each category.

Date ____________________ Dr. ____________________

Medical Facility ____________________

City ____________________ State ____________________

Phone (______) ____________________ Other ____________________

Temperature ____________________ Blood pressure ____________________

Pulse ____________________ Glucose ____________________

Other ____________________

Blood Test ____________________

Anesthesia ____________________ Dr. ____________________

Reaction: ❑ No ❑ Yes ____________________

____

____

Counteraction ____________________

____

____

Procedure ____________________

____

____

Summary ____________________

____

____

Complications ____________________

____

Length of Stay ____________________

____

❑ *See hospital discharge and care instructions.*

Add a separate page if you need to write more detail.

Hospitalizations * Surgeries * Procedures Records

❑ **HOSPITALIZATION** ❑ **SURGERY** ❑ **PROCEDURE**

Best to use a separate page for each category.

Date ______________ Dr. ______________________________

Medical Facility ______________________________

City ______________________ State ______________________

Phone (   ) ______________________ Other ______________________

Temperature ______________________ Blood pressure ______________________

Pulse ______________________ Glucose ______________________

Other ______________________________

Blood Test ______________________________

Anesthesia ______________________ Dr. ______________________

Reaction: ❑ No ❑ Yes ______________________________

____

____

Counteraction ______________________________

____

____

Procedure ______________________________

____

____

Summary ______________________________

____

____

Complications ______________________________

____

Length of Stay ______________________________

____

❑ *See hospital discharge and care instructions.*

Add a separate page if you need to write more detail.

Hospitalizations * Surgeries * Procedures Records

❑ **HOSPITALIZATION** ❑ **SURGERY** ❑ **PROCEDURE**

Best to use a separate page for each category.

Date ____________________ Dr. ____________________

Medical Facility ____________________

City ____________________ State ____________________

Phone (______) ____________________ Other ____________________

Temperature ____________________ Blood pressure ____________________

Pulse ____________________ Glucose ____________________

Other ____________________

Blood Test ____________________

Anesthesia ____________________ Dr. ____________________

Reaction: ❑ No ❑ Yes ____________________

____

____

Counteraction ____________________

____

____

Procedure ____________________

____

____

Summary ____________________

____

____

Complications ____________________

____

Length of Stay ____________________

____

❑ *See hospital discharge and care instructions.*

Add a separate page if you need to write more detail.

Hospitalizations * Surgeries * Procedures Records

❑ **HOSPITALIZATION** ❑ **SURGERY** ❑ **PROCEDURE**

Best to use a separate page for each category.

Date ____________ Dr. ____________

Medical Facility ____________

City ____________ State ____________

Phone (   ) ____________ Other ____________

Temperature ____________ Blood pressure ____________

Pulse ____________ Glucose ____________

Other ____________

Blood Test ____________

Anesthesia ____________ Dr. ____________

Reaction: ❑ No ❑ Yes ____________

Counteraction ____________

Procedure ____________

Summary ____________

Complications ____________

Length of Stay ____________

❑ *See hospital discharge and care instructions.*

Add a separate page if you need to write more detail.

Hospitalizations * Surgeries * Procedures Records

❑ **HOSPITALIZATION** ❑ **SURGERY** ❑ **PROCEDURE**

Best to use a separate page for each category.

Date ____________________ Dr. ____________________

Medical Facility ____________________

City ____________________ State ____________________

Phone (   ) ____________________ Other ____________________

Temperature ____________________ Blood pressure ____________________

Pulse ____________________ Glucose ____________________

Other ____________________

Blood Test ____________________

Anesthesia ____________________ Dr. ____________________

Reaction: ❑ No ❑ Yes ____________________

____

____

Counteraction ____________________

____

____

Procedure ____________________

____

____

Summary ____________________

____

____

Complications ____________________

____

Length of Stay ____________________

____

❑ *See hospital discharge and care instructions.*

Add a separate page if you need to write more detail.

Hospitalizations * Surgeries * Procedures Records

❑ **HOSPITALIZATION** ❑ **SURGERY** ❑ **PROCEDURE**

Best to use a separate page for each category.

Date ____________ Dr. ____________

Medical Facility ____________

City ____________ State ____________

Phone ( ) ____________ Other ____________

Temperature ____________ Blood pressure ____________

Pulse ____________ Glucose ____________

Other ____________

Blood Test ____________

Anesthesia ____________ Dr. ____________

Reaction: ❑ No ❑ Yes ____________

Counteraction ____________

Procedure ____________

Summary ____________

Complications ____________

Length of Stay ____________

❑ *See hospital discharge and care instructions.*

Add a separate page if you need to write more detail.

Hospitalizations * Surgeries * Procedures Records

❑ **HOSPITALIZATION** ❑ **SURGERY** ❑ **PROCEDURE**

Best to use a separate page for each category.

Date ____________________ Dr. ____

Medical Facility ____

City ______________________________ State ______________________________

Phone (   ) ________________________ Other ______________________________

Temperature __________________________ Blood pressure __________________________

Pulse ______________________________ Glucose ______________________________

Other ____

Blood Test ____

Anesthesia ____________________________ Dr. ______________________________

Reaction: ❑ No ❑ Yes ____

____

____

Counteraction ____

____

____

Procedure ____

____

____

Summary ____

____

____

Complications ____

____

Length of Stay ____

____

❑ *See hospital discharge and care instructions.*

Add a separate page if you need to write more detail.

Hospitalizations * Surgeries * Procedures Records

❑ **HOSPITALIZATION** ❑ **SURGERY** ❑ **PROCEDURE**

Best to use a separate page for each category.

Date ____________ Dr. ____________

Medical Facility ____________

City ____________ State ____________

Phone (   ) ____________ Other ____________

Temperature ____________ Blood pressure ____________

Pulse ____________ Glucose ____________

Other ____________

Blood Test ____________

Anesthesia ____________ Dr. ____________

Reaction: ❑ No ❑ Yes ____________

Counteraction ____________

Procedure ____________

Summary ____________

Complications ____________

Length of Stay ____________

❑ *See hospital discharge and care instructions.*

Add a separate page if you need to write more detail.

Medical * Doctor Appointments Log and Records

Log

Maintain a log for easy recall and review.

Records

Write down the reason for the visit, specify if it is routine or an emergency, etc. This is especially helpful to keep abreast of what has occurred, and for a continuum of health. You can have the doctor summarize the procedure, complications, and any notes in this area. If, you consider this information beneficial, ask for a copy of the doctor's report for your file or binder.

You will find a section on "Questions to Ask Your Doctor" (pages 16-18). This will help you compile a list of questions and concerns that you will want to ask and inform your doctor at the time of your appointment.

Notes

Medical * Doctor Appointment Log

Maintain a log for easy recall and review.

Date	Doctor	Purpose

Medical * Doctor Appointment Log

Maintain a log for easy recall and review.

Date	Doctor	Purpose

Medical * Doctor Appointment Records

❑ **DOCTOR VISITS** ❑ **OTHER SERVICES** ❑ **THERAPISTS**

Best to use a separate page for each category. Year ____________

Date ____________________ Dr. / Other ____

Purpose ____

____

Temperature ______________ Blood Pressure ________________ Pulse ________________

Glucose _________________ Other _______________________ Weight _______________

Blood Test ____

❑ Lab ❑ X-ray ❑ Other Tests ____

❑ Special Referral Dr. / Other Tests ____

Phone (   ) ____ ❑ Referral Slip ❑ X-ray Copy

Purpose ____

____

____

Next Appointment Date ______________________________ Time ____________________

❑ Request copy of Dr.'s report sent to Home and ❑ Other __________________________

Visit Summary ____

____

____

QUESTIONS - CONCERNS

It is always helpful to have your list ready before your appointment.

____

____

____

____

____

____

____

____

Medical * Doctor Appointment Records

❑ **DOCTOR VISITS** ❑ **OTHER SERVICES** ❑ **THERAPISTS**

Best to use a separate page for each category. Year ______________

Date ______________________ Dr. / Other ____

Purpose ____

____

Temperature _______________ Blood Pressure __________________ Pulse ____________________

Glucose ___________________ Other _________________________ Weight ___________________

Blood Test ____

❑ Lab ❑ X-ray ❑ Other Tests ____

❑ Special Referral Dr. / Other Tests ____

Phone (   ) _____________________________________ ❑ Referral Slip ❑ X-ray Copy

Purpose ____

____

____

Next Appointment Date ________________________________ Time ____________________

❑ Request copy of Dr.'s report sent to Home and ❑ Other ______________________________

Visit Summary ____

____

____

QUESTIONS - CONCERNS

It is always helpful to have your list ready before your appointment.

____

____

____

____

____

____

____

____

Medical * Doctor Appointment Records

❑ **DOCTOR VISITS** ❑ **OTHER SERVICES** ❑ **THERAPISTS**

Best to use a separate page for each category. Year ____________

Date ____________________ Dr. / Other ______________________________

Purpose ____

____

Temperature ____________ Blood Pressure ______________ Pulse ____________

Glucose ________________ Other ____________________ Weight ____________

Blood Test ____

❑ Lab ❑ X-ray ❑ Other Tests ______________________________________

❑ Special Referral Dr. / Other Tests _________________________________

Phone (   ) ______________________________ ❑ Referral Slip ❑ X-ray Copy

Purpose ____

____

____

Next Appointment Date ______________________________ Time ____________

❑ Request copy of Dr.'s report sent to Home and ❑ Other ____________________

Visit Summary ____

____

____

QUESTIONS - CONCERNS

It is always helpful to have your list ready before your appointment.

____

____

____

____

____

____

____

____

Medical * Doctor Appointment Records

❑ **DOCTOR VISITS** ❑ **OTHER SERVICES** ❑ **THERAPISTS**

Best to use a separate page for each category. Year ______________

Date ______________________ Dr. / Other ____

Purpose ____

____

Temperature ______________ Blood Pressure __________________ Pulse ____________________

Glucose ___________________ Other _________________________ Weight ___________________

Blood Test ____

❑ Lab ❑ X-ray ❑ Other Tests ____

❑ Special Referral Dr. / Other Tests ____

Phone (   ) ____ ❑ Referral Slip ❑ X-ray Copy

Purpose ____

____

____

Next Appointment Date ________________________________ Time ___________________________

❑ Request copy of Dr.'s report sent to Home and ❑ Other _____________________________

Visit Summary ____

____

____

QUESTIONS - CONCERNS

It is always helpful to have your list ready before your appointment.

____

____

____

____

____

____

____

____

Medical * Doctor Appointment Records

❑ **DOCTOR VISITS** ❑ **OTHER SERVICES** ❑ **THERAPISTS**

Best to use a separate page for each category. Year ____________

Date ____________________ Dr. / Other ______________________________

Purpose ____

____

Temperature ____________ Blood Pressure ______________ Pulse ____________

Glucose ________________ Other ______________________ Weight ____________

Blood Test ____

❑ Lab ❑ X-ray ❑ Other Tests ____________________________________

❑ Special Referral Dr. / Other Tests ______________________________

Phone (   ) ____________________________ ❑ Referral Slip ❑ X-ray Copy

Purpose ____

____

____

Next Appointment Date ____________________________ Time ______________

❑ Request copy of Dr.'s report sent to Home and ❑ Other _______________

Visit Summary ____

____

____

QUESTIONS - CONCERNS

It is always helpful to have your list ready before your appointment.

____

____

____

____

____

____

____

____

Medical * Doctor Appointment Records

❑ **DOCTOR VISITS** ❑ **OTHER SERVICES** ❑ **THERAPISTS**

Best to use a separate page for each category. Year ____________

Date ____________________ Dr. / Other ____

Purpose ____

____

Temperature ____________ Blood Pressure ________________ Pulse ______________

Glucose ________________ Other ______________________ Weight ______________

Blood Test ____

❑ Lab ❑ X-ray ❑ Other Tests ____

❑ Special Referral Dr. / Other Tests ______________________________________

Phone (   ) ________________________________ ❑ Referral Slip ❑ X-ray Copy

Purpose ____

____

____

Next Appointment Date ____________________________ Time ____________________

❑ Request copy of Dr.'s report sent to Home and ❑ Other ______________________

Visit Summary ____

____

____

QUESTIONS - CONCERNS

It is always helpful to have your list ready before your appointment.

____

____

____

____

____

____

____

____

Medical * Doctor Appointment Records

❑ **DOCTOR VISITS** ❑ **OTHER SERVICES** ❑ **THERAPISTS**

Best to use a separate page for each category. Year ____________

Date ____________________ Dr. / Other ____

Purpose ____

____

Temperature ______________ Blood Pressure ________________ Pulse __________________

Glucose _________________ Other _______________________ Weight _________________

Blood Test ____

❑ Lab ❑ X-ray ❑ Other Tests ____

❑ Special Referral Dr. / Other Tests ____

Phone (   ) _____________________________________ ❑ Referral Slip ❑ X-ray Copy

Purpose ____

____

____

Next Appointment Date _____________________________ Time __________________

❑ Request copy of Dr.'s report sent to Home and ❑ Other _______________________

Visit Summary ____

____

____

QUESTIONS - CONCERNS

It is always helpful to have your list ready before your appointment.

____

____

____

____

____

____

____

____

Medical * Doctor Appointment Records

❑ **DOCTOR VISITS** ❑ **OTHER SERVICES** ❑ **THERAPISTS**

Best to use a separate page for each category. Year ______________

Date ______________________ Dr. / Other ____

Purpose ____

____

Temperature _______________ Blood Pressure __________________ Pulse ____________________

Glucose ___________________ Other __________________________ Weight ___________________

Blood Test ____

❑ Lab ❑ X-ray ❑ Other Tests ____

❑ Special Referral Dr. / Other Tests ____

Phone (   ) ____ ❑ Referral Slip ❑ X-ray Copy

Purpose ____

____

____

Next Appointment Date ________________________________ Time ___________________________

❑ Request copy of Dr.'s report sent to Home and ❑ Other ______________________________________

Visit Summary ____

____

____

QUESTIONS - CONCERNS

It is always helpful to have your list ready before your appointment.

____

____

____

____

____

____

____

____

Medical * Doctor Appointment Records

❑ **DOCTOR VISITS** ❑ **OTHER SERVICES** ❑ **THERAPISTS**

Best to use a separate page for each category. Year ______

Date ______ Dr. / Other ______

Purpose ______

______

Temperature ______ Blood Pressure ______ Pulse ______

Glucose ______ Other ______ Weight ______

Blood Test ______

❑ Lab ❑ X-ray ❑ Other Tests ______

❑ Special Referral Dr. / Other Tests ______

Phone ( ) ______ ❑ Referral Slip ❑ X-ray Copy

Purpose ______

______

______

Next Appointment Date ______ Time ______

❑ Request copy of Dr.'s report sent to Home and ❑ Other ______

Visit Summary ______

______

______

QUESTIONS - CONCERNS

It is always helpful to have your list ready before your appointment.

______

______

______

______

______

______

______

______

Medical * Doctor Appointment Records

❑ **DOCTOR VISITS** ❑ **OTHER SERVICES** ❑ **THERAPISTS**

Best to use a separate page for each category. Year ____________

Date ____________________ Dr. / Other ____

Purpose ____

____

Temperature ______________ Blood Pressure ________________ Pulse ________________

Glucose __________________ Other ______________________ Weight ________________

Blood Test ____

❑ Lab ❑ X-ray ❑ Other Tests ____

❑ Special Referral Dr. / Other Tests ______________________________________

Phone (   ) ____________________________________ ❑ Referral Slip ❑ X-ray Copy

Purpose ____

____

____

Next Appointment Date ______________________________ Time ________________

❑ Request copy of Dr.'s report sent to Home and ❑ Other ________________________

Visit Summary ____

____

____

QUESTIONS - CONCERNS

It is always helpful to have your list ready before your appointment.

____

____

____

____

____

____

____

____

Medical * Doctor Appointment Records

❑ **DOCTOR VISITS** ❑ **OTHER SERVICES** ❑ **THERAPISTS**

Best to use a separate page for each category. Year ____________

Date ____________________ Dr. / Other ________________________________

Purpose ____

____

Temperature ______________ Blood Pressure ________________ Pulse __________________

Glucose __________________ Other _______________________ Weight _________________

Blood Test ____

❑ Lab ❑ X-ray ❑ Other Tests ____

❑ Special Referral Dr. / Other Tests ___________________________________

Phone (   ) ________________________________ ❑ Referral Slip ❑ X-ray Copy

Purpose ____

____

____

Next Appointment Date ______________________________ Time ____________________

❑ Request copy of Dr.'s report sent to Home and ❑ Other ______________________

Visit Summary ____

____

____

QUESTIONS - CONCERNS

It is always helpful to have your list ready before your appointment.

____

____

____

____

____

____

____

____

Medical * Doctor Appointment Records

❑ **DOCTOR VISITS** ❑ **OTHER SERVICES** ❑ **THERAPISTS**

Best to use a separate page for each category. Year ____________

Date ____________________ Dr. / Other ________________________________

Purpose ____

____

Temperature ______________ Blood Pressure ________________ Pulse ______________

Glucose ________________ Other ______________________ Weight ______________

Blood Test ____

❑ Lab ❑ X-ray ❑ Other Tests ____

❑ Special Referral Dr. / Other Tests ______________________________________

Phone (   ) ______________________________________ ❑ Referral Slip ❑ X-ray Copy

Purpose ____

____

____

Next Appointment Date ___________________________ Time _______________________

❑ Request copy of Dr.'s report sent to Home and ❑ Other ______________________

Visit Summary ____

____

____

QUESTIONS - CONCERNS

It is always helpful to have your list ready before your appointment.

____

____

____

____

____

____

____

____

Medical * Doctor Appointment Records

❑ **DOCTOR VISITS** ❑ **OTHER SERVICES** ❑ **THERAPISTS**

Best to use a separate page for each category. Year ____________

Date ____________________ Dr. / Other ____

Purpose ____

____

Temperature ______________ Blood Pressure _________________ Pulse ________________

Glucose __________________ Other _________________________ Weight _______________

Blood Test ____

❑ Lab ❑ X-ray ❑ Other Tests ____

❑ Special Referral Dr. / Other Tests ____

Phone (______) ____ ❑ Referral Slip ❑ X-ray Copy

Purpose ____

____

____

Next Appointment Date _______________________________ Time ________________

❑ Request copy of Dr.'s report sent to Home and ❑ Other ________________________

Visit Summary ____

____

____

QUESTIONS - CONCERNS

It is always helpful to have your list ready before your appointment.

____

____

____

____

____

____

____

____

Medical * Doctor Appointment Records

❑ **DOCTOR VISITS** ❑ **OTHER SERVICES** ❑ **THERAPISTS**

Best to use a separate page for each category. Year ____________

Date ____________________ Dr. / Other ______________________________

Purpose ____

____

Temperature ____________ Blood Pressure ______________ Pulse ______________

Glucose ______________ Other ____________________ Weight ______________

Blood Test ____

❑ Lab ❑ X-ray ❑ Other Tests ____

❑ Special Referral Dr. / Other Tests ______________________________________

Phone (   ) ______________________________ ❑ Referral Slip ❑ X-ray Copy

Purpose ____

____

____

Next Appointment Date ________________________ Time ________________

❑ Request copy of Dr.'s report sent to Home and ❑ Other ________________________

Visit Summary ____

____

____

QUESTIONS - CONCERNS

It is always helpful to have your list ready before your appointment.

____

____

____

____

____

____

____

____

Medical * Doctor Appointment Records

❑ **DOCTOR VISITS** ❑ **OTHER SERVICES** ❑ **THERAPISTS**

Best to use a separate page for each category. Year ____________

Date ____________________ Dr. / Other ______________________________

Purpose ____

____

Temperature ____________ Blood Pressure ______________ Pulse ____________

Glucose ______________ Other ____________________ Weight _____________

Blood Test ____

❑ Lab ❑ X-ray ❑ Other Tests ___________________________________

❑ Special Referral Dr. / Other Tests ______________________________

Phone (______) ________________________________ ❑ Referral Slip ❑ X-ray Copy

Purpose ____

____

____

Next Appointment Date ___________________________ Time ______________

❑ Request copy of Dr.'s report sent to Home and ❑ Other ________________

Visit Summary ____

____

____

QUESTIONS - CONCERNS

It is always helpful to have your list ready before your appointment.

____

____

____

____

____

____

____

____

Medical * Doctor Appointment Records

❑ **DOCTOR VISITS** ❑ **OTHER SERVICES** ❑ **THERAPISTS**

Best to use a separate page for each category. Year ____________

Date ____________________ Dr. / Other ______________________________

Purpose ____

____

Temperature ____________ Blood Pressure ____________ Pulse ____________

Glucose ____________ Other ____________ Weight ____________

Blood Test ____

❑ Lab ❑ X-ray ❑ Other Tests ______________________________

❑ Special Referral Dr. / Other Tests ______________________________

Phone (   ) ______________________________ ❑ Referral Slip ❑ X-ray Copy

Purpose ____

____

____

Next Appointment Date ____________________ Time ____________

❑ Request copy of Dr.'s report sent to Home and ❑ Other ____________________

Visit Summary ____

____

____

QUESTIONS - CONCERNS

It is always helpful to have your list ready before your appointment.

____

____

____

____

____

____

____

____

Medical * Doctor Appointment Records

❑ **DOCTOR VISITS** ❑ **OTHER SERVICES** ❑ **THERAPISTS**

Best to use a separate page for each category. Year ____________

Date ____________________ Dr. / Other ____

Purpose ____

____

Temperature ____________ Blood Pressure ______________ Pulse ______________

Glucose ________________ Other ____________________ Weight ______________

Blood Test ____

❑ Lab ❑ X-ray ❑ Other Tests ____

❑ Special Referral Dr. / Other Tests ____________________________________

Phone (   ) ____ ❑ Referral Slip ❑ X-ray Copy

Purpose ____

____

____

Next Appointment Date ____________________________ Time ______________________

❑ Request copy of Dr.'s report sent to Home and ❑ Other ____________________________

Visit Summary ____

____

____

QUESTIONS - CONCERNS

It is always helpful to have your list ready before your appointment.

____

____

____

____

____

____

____

____

Medical * Doctor Appointment Records

❑ **DOCTOR VISITS** ❑ **OTHER SERVICES** ❑ **THERAPISTS**

Best to use a separate page for each category. Year ____________

Date ____________________ Dr. / Other ____

Purpose ____

____

Temperature ______________ Blood Pressure ________________ Pulse ______________

Glucose __________________ Other ______________________ Weight ______________

Blood Test ____

❑ Lab ❑ X-ray ❑ Other Tests ____

❑ Special Referral Dr. / Other Tests _______________________________________

Phone (   ) _____________________________ ❑ Referral Slip ❑ X-ray Copy

Purpose ____

____

____

Next Appointment Date _____________________________ Time ________________

❑ Request copy of Dr.'s report sent to Home and ❑ Other _______________________

Visit Summary ____

____

____

QUESTIONS - CONCERNS

It is always helpful to have your list ready before your appointment.

____

____

____

____

____

____

____

____

Medical * Doctor Appointment Records

❑ **DOCTOR VISITS** ❑ **OTHER SERVICES** ❑ **THERAPISTS**

Best to use a separate page for each category. Year ______________

Date ______________________ Dr. / Other ____

Purpose ____

____

Temperature _______________ Blood Pressure __________________ Pulse ____________________

Glucose ___________________ Other __________________________ Weight ___________________

Blood Test ____

❑ Lab ❑ X-ray ❑ Other Tests ____

❑ Special Referral Dr. / Other Tests ____

Phone (   ) ____ ❑ Referral Slip ❑ X-ray Copy

Purpose ____

____

____

Next Appointment Date _________________________________ Time __________________________

❑ Request copy of Dr.'s report sent to Home and ❑ Other ____________________________________

Visit Summary ____

____

____

QUESTIONS - CONCERNS

It is always helpful to have your list ready before your appointment.

____

____

____

____

____

____

____

____

Medical * Doctor Appointment Records

❑ **DOCTOR VISITS** ❑ **OTHER SERVICES** ❑ **THERAPISTS**

Best to use a separate page for each category. Year ____________

Date ____________________ Dr. / Other ____

Purpose ____

____

Temperature ____________ Blood Pressure ______________ Pulse ______________

Glucose ________________ Other ____________________ Weight ______________

Blood Test ____

❑ Lab ❑ X-ray ❑ Other Tests ____

❑ Special Referral Dr. / Other Tests ____________________________________

Phone (   ) ____ ❑ Referral Slip ❑ X-ray Copy

Purpose ____

____

____

Next Appointment Date ____________________________ Time ____________________

❑ Request copy of Dr.'s report sent to Home and ❑ Other ______________________

Visit Summary ____

____

____

QUESTIONS - CONCERNS

It is always helpful to have your list ready before your appointment.

____

____

____

____

____

____

____

____

Medical * Doctor Appointment Records

❑ **DOCTOR VISITS** ❑ **OTHER SERVICES** ❑ **THERAPISTS**

Best to use a separate page for each category. Year ______________

Date ______________________ Dr. / Other ____

Purpose ____

____

Temperature _______________ Blood Pressure _________________ Pulse ____________________

Glucose ___________________ Other _________________________ Weight __________________

Blood Test ____

❑ Lab ❑ X-ray ❑ Other Tests ____

❑ Special Referral Dr. / Other Tests ____

Phone ( ) ____ ❑ Referral Slip ❑ X-ray Copy

Purpose ____

____

____

Next Appointment Date ________________________________ Time ______________________

❑ Request copy of Dr.'s report sent to Home and ❑ Other _______________________________

Visit Summary ____

____

____

QUESTIONS - CONCERNS

It is always helpful to have your list ready before your appointment.

____

____

____

____

____

____

____

____

Medical * Doctor Appointment Records

❑ **DOCTOR VISITS** ❑ **OTHER SERVICES** ❑ **THERAPISTS**

Best to use a separate page for each category. Year ____________

Date ____________________ Dr. / Other ____

Purpose ____

____

Temperature ______________ Blood Pressure ________________ Pulse __________________

Glucose _________________ Other ______________________ Weight _________________

Blood Test ____

❑ Lab ❑ X-ray ❑ Other Tests ____

❑ Special Referral Dr. / Other Tests ____

Phone ( ) ______________________________________ ❑ Referral Slip ❑ X-ray Copy

Purpose ____

____

____

Next Appointment Date ____________________________ Time ______________________

❑ Request copy of Dr.'s report sent to Home and ❑ Other __________________________

Visit Summary ____

____

____

QUESTIONS - CONCERNS

It is always helpful to have your list ready before your appointment.

____

____

____

____

____

____

____

____

Medical * Doctor Appointment Records

❑ **DOCTOR VISITS** ❑ **OTHER SERVICES** ❑ **THERAPISTS**

Best to use a separate page for each category. Year ____________

Date ____________________ Dr. / Other ______________________________________

Purpose ____

____

Temperature ______________ Blood Pressure ________________ Pulse __________________

Glucose __________________ Other _______________________ Weight _________________

Blood Test ____

❑ Lab ❑ X-ray ❑ Other Tests ____

❑ Special Referral Dr. / Other Tests ____

Phone (   ) _____________________________________ ❑ Referral Slip ❑ X-ray Copy

Purpose ____

____

____

Next Appointment Date ______________________________ Time _________________

❑ Request copy of Dr.'s report sent to Home and ❑ Other _____________________________

Visit Summary ____

____

____

QUESTIONS - CONCERNS

It is always helpful to have your list ready before your appointment.

____

____

____

____

____

____

____

____

Medical * Doctor Appointment Records

❑ **DOCTOR VISITS** ❑ **OTHER SERVICES** ❑ **THERAPISTS**

Best to use a separate page for each category. Year ______________

Date ______________________ Dr. / Other ____

Purpose ____

____

Temperature _______________ Blood Pressure __________________ Pulse ____________________

Glucose ___________________ Other _________________________ Weight ___________________

Blood Test ____

❑ Lab ❑ X-ray ❑ Other Tests ____

❑ Special Referral Dr. / Other Tests ____

Phone (   ) ____ ❑ Referral Slip ❑ X-ray Copy

Purpose ____

____

____

Next Appointment Date ________________________________ Time _____________________________

❑ Request copy of Dr.'s report sent to Home and ❑ Other ____

Visit Summary ____

____

____

QUESTIONS - CONCERNS

It is always helpful to have your list ready before your appointment.

____

____

____

____

____

____

____

____

Medical * Doctor Appointment Records

❑ **DOCTOR VISITS** ❑ **OTHER SERVICES** ❑ **THERAPISTS**

Best to use a separate page for each category. Year ____________

Date ____________________ Dr. / Other ____

Purpose ____

____

Temperature ______________ Blood Pressure ________________ Pulse ________________

Glucose _________________ Other _______________________ Weight _________________

Blood Test ____

❑ Lab ❑ X-ray ❑ Other Tests ____

❑ Special Referral Dr. / Other Tests ____

Phone (   ) _____________________________________ ❑ Referral Slip ❑ X-ray Copy

Purpose ____

____

____

Next Appointment Date _____________________________ Time _________________

❑ Request copy of Dr.'s report sent to Home and ❑ Other ____________________________

Visit Summary ____

____

____

QUESTIONS - CONCERNS

It is always helpful to have your list ready before your appointment.

____

____

____

____

____

____

____

____

Medical * Doctor Appointment Records

❑ **DOCTOR VISITS** ❑ **OTHER SERVICES** ❑ **THERAPISTS**

Best to use a separate page for each category. Year ____________

Date ____________________ Dr. / Other ______________________________

Purpose ____

____

Temperature ____________ Blood Pressure ______________ Pulse ______________

Glucose ______________ Other ____________________ Weight ______________

Blood Test ____

❑ Lab ❑ X-ray ❑ Other Tests ________________________________

❑ Special Referral Dr. / Other Tests ______________________________

Phone (   ) ______________________________ ❑ Referral Slip ❑ X-ray Copy

Purpose ____

____

____

Next Appointment Date ________________________ Time ______________

❑ Request copy of Dr.'s report sent to Home and ❑ Other ______________________

Visit Summary ____

____

____

QUESTIONS - CONCERNS

It is always helpful to have your list ready before your appointment.

____

____

____

____

____

____

____

____

Medical * Doctor Appointment Records

❑ **DOCTOR VISITS** ❑ **OTHER SERVICES** ❑ **THERAPISTS**

Best to use a separate page for each category. Year ____________

Date ____________________ Dr. / Other ____

Purpose ____

____

Temperature ______________ Blood Pressure ________________ Pulse __________________

Glucose __________________ Other _______________________ Weight _________________

Blood Test ____

❑ Lab ❑ X-ray ❑ Other Tests ____

❑ Special Referral Dr. / Other Tests ____

Phone (   ) ____ ❑ Referral Slip ❑ X-ray Copy

Purpose ____

____

____

Next Appointment Date _____________________________ Time ________________________

❑ Request copy of Dr.'s report sent to Home and ❑ Other ___________________________________

Visit Summary ____

____

____

QUESTIONS - CONCERNS

It is always helpful to have your list ready before your appointment.

____

____

____

____

____

____

____

____

Medical * Doctor Appointment Records

❑ **DOCTOR VISITS** ❑ **OTHER SERVICES** ❑ **THERAPISTS**

Best to use a separate page for each category. Year ____________

Date ____________________ Dr. / Other ____

Purpose ____

____

Temperature ______________ Blood Pressure ________________ Pulse ________________

Glucose _________________ Other _______________________ Weight ________________

Blood Test ____

❑ Lab ❑ X-ray ❑ Other Tests ____

❑ Special Referral Dr. / Other Tests ____

Phone (   ) ____________________________________ ❑ Referral Slip ❑ X-ray Copy

Purpose ____

____

____

Next Appointment Date ____________________________ Time ____________________

❑ Request copy of Dr.'s report sent to Home and ❑ Other ___________________________

Visit Summary ____

____

____

QUESTIONS - CONCERNS

It is always helpful to have your list ready before your appointment.

____

____

____

____

____

____

____

____

Medical * Doctor Appointment Records

❑ **DOCTOR VISITS** ❑ **OTHER SERVICES** ❑ **THERAPISTS**

Best to use a separate page for each category. Year ____________

Date ____________________ Dr. / Other ____

Purpose ____

____

Temperature ______________ Blood Pressure ________________ Pulse __________________

Glucose __________________ Other _______________________ Weight _________________

Blood Test ____

❑ Lab ❑ X-ray ❑ Other Tests ____

❑ Special Referral Dr. / Other Tests ____

Phone (_____) ______________________________________ ❑ Referral Slip ❑ X-ray Copy

Purpose ____

____

____

Next Appointment Date ____________________________ Time _________________________

❑ Request copy of Dr.'s report sent to Home and ❑ Other _____________________________

Visit Summary ____

____

____

QUESTIONS - CONCERNS

It is always helpful to have your list ready before your appointment.

____

____

____

____

____

____

____

____

Medical * Doctor Appointment Records

❑ **DOCTOR VISITS** ❑ **OTHER SERVICES** ❑ **THERAPISTS**

Best to use a separate page for each category. Year ____________

Date ____________________ Dr. / Other ______________________________

Purpose ____

____

Temperature ____________ Blood Pressure ____________ Pulse ____________

Glucose ____________ Other ____________ Weight ____________

Blood Test ____

❑ Lab ❑ X-ray ❑ Other Tests ______________________________

❑ Special Referral Dr. / Other Tests ______________________________

Phone (   ) ______________________________ ❑ Referral Slip ❑ X-ray Copy

Purpose ____

____

____

Next Appointment Date ____________________ Time ____________

❑ Request copy of Dr.'s report sent to Home and ❑ Other ____________________

Visit Summary ____

____

____

QUESTIONS - CONCERNS

It is always helpful to have your list ready before your appointment.

____

____

____

____

____

____

____

____

Dental Appointments Log and Records

Log

Maintain a log for easy recall and review.

Records

Write down the reason for the visit, specify if it is routine or an emergency, etc. This is especially helpful to keep abreast of what has occurred, and for a continuum of health. You can have the dentist summarize the procedure, complications, and any notes in this area. If, you consider this information beneficial, ask for a copy of the doctor's report for your file or binder.

You will find a section on "Questions to Ask Your Doctor" (pages 16-18). This will help you compile a list of questions and concerns that you will want to ask and inform your doctor at the time of your appointment.

Notes

Dental Appointment Log

Maintain a log for easy recall and review.

Date	Doctor	Purpose
		❒ Cleaning
		❒ Cleaning
		❒ Cleaning
		❒ Cleaning
		❒ Cleaning
		❒ Cleaning
		❒ Cleaning
		❒ Cleaning
		❒ Cleaning
		❒ Cleaning
		❒ Cleaning
		❒ Cleaning
		❒ Cleaning
		❒ Cleaning
		❒ Cleaning
		❒ Cleaning

Dental Appointment Log

Maintain a log for easy recall and review.

Date	Doctor	Purpose

Dental Appointment Records

❑ **DOCTOR VISITS** ❑ **OTHER SERVICES**

Best to use a separate page for each category. Year ____________

Date ____________________ Dr. / Other ____

Purpose ____

____

Treatment Plan ______________ ❑ Pending ❑ Type ______________________________

Treatment Summary ____

❑ Lab ❑ X-ray ❑ Dental Impressions Type ______________________________________

Next Appointment Date ______________________________ Time ______________

❑ Request copy of Dr.'s report sent to Home and ❑ Other ______________________________

❑ Special Referral Dr. / Other ____

Phone (______) ____________________________________ ❑ Referral Slip ❑ X-ray Copy

Purpose ____

____

Visit Summary ____

____

____

____

QUESTIONS - CONCERNS

It is always helpful to have your list ready before your appointment.

____

____

____

____

____

____

____

____

____

Dental Appointment Records

❑ **DOCTOR VISITS** ❑ **OTHER SERVICES**

Best to use a separate page for each category. Year ____________

Date ____________________ Dr. / Other ____

Purpose ____

____

Treatment Plan ______________ ❑ Pending ❑ Type ______________________________

Treatment Summary ____

❑ Lab ❑ X-ray ❑ Dental Impressions Type ______________________________________

Next Appointment Date ______________________________ Time ______________________

❑ Request copy of Dr.'s report sent to Home and ❑ Other _____________________________

❑ Special Referral Dr. / Other ____

Phone (   ) ______________________________ ❑ Referral Slip ❑ X-ray Copy

Purpose ____

____

Visit Summary ____

____

____

____

QUESTIONS - CONCERNS
It is always helpful to have your list ready before your appointment.

____

____

____

____

____

____

____

____

____

Dental Appointment Records

❑ **DOCTOR VISITS** ❑ **OTHER SERVICES**

Best to use a separate page for each category. Year ____________

Date ____________________ Dr. / Other ____

Purpose ____

____

Treatment Plan ______________ ❑ Pending ❑ Type ____________________________

Treatment Summary ____

❑ Lab ❑ X-ray ❑ Dental Impressions Type ____________________________________

Next Appointment Date ______________________________ Time ________________

❑ Request copy of Dr.'s report sent to Home and ❑ Other _______________________

❑ Special Referral Dr. / Other ____

Phone (______) ____________________________________ ❑ Referral Slip ❑ X-ray Copy

Purpose ____

____

Visit Summary ____

____

____

____

QUESTIONS - CONCERNS
It is always helpful to have your list ready before your appointment.

____

____

____

____

____

____

____

____

____

Dental Appointments

Dental Appointment Records

❑ **DOCTOR VISITS** ❑ **OTHER SERVICES**

Best to use a separate page for each category. Year ____________

Date ____________________ Dr. / Other ____

Purpose ____

____

Treatment Plan ______________ ❑ Pending ❑ Type ________________________________

Treatment Summary ____

❑ Lab ❑ X-ray ❑ Dental Impressions Type ____

Next Appointment Date ______________________________ Time ______________________

❑ Request copy of Dr.'s report sent to Home and ❑ Other ________________________________

❑ Special Referral Dr. / Other ____

Phone (   ) ______________________________________ ❑ Referral Slip ❑ X-ray Copy

Purpose ____

____

Visit Summary ____

____

____

____

QUESTIONS - CONCERNS
It is always helpful to have your list ready before your appointment.

____

____

____

____

____

____

____

____

____

Dental Appointment Records

❑ **DOCTOR VISITS** ❑ **OTHER SERVICES**

Best to use a separate page for each category. Year ____________

Date ____________________ Dr. / Other ________________________________

Purpose ____

____

Treatment Plan ______________ ❑ Pending ❑ Type ______________________

Treatment Summary ______________________________________

❑ Lab ❑ X-ray ❑ Dental Impressions Type ______________________

Next Appointment Date ______________________ Time ______________

❑ Request copy of Dr.'s report sent to Home and ❑ Other ______________

❑ Special Referral Dr. / Other __________________________________

Phone (______) ______________________ ❑ Referral Slip ❑ X-ray Copy

Purpose ____

____

Visit Summary ____

____

____

____

QUESTIONS - CONCERNS
It is always helpful to have your list ready before your appointment.

____

____

____

____

____

____

____

____

____

Dental Appointments

Dental Appointment Records

❑ **DOCTOR VISITS** ❑ **OTHER SERVICES**

Best to use a separate page for each category. Year ____________

Date ____________________ Dr. / Other ____

Purpose ____

____

Treatment Plan ______________ ❑ Pending ❑ Type ________________________________

Treatment Summary ____

❑ Lab ❑ X-ray ❑ Dental Impressions Type ____

Next Appointment Date ______________________________ Time ______________________

❑ Request copy of Dr.'s report sent to Home and ❑ Other _________________________________

❑ Special Referral Dr. / Other ____

Phone (   ) ____ ❑ Referral Slip ❑ X-ray Copy

Purpose ____

____

Visit Summary ____

____

____

____

QUESTIONS - CONCERNS
It is always helpful to have your list ready before your appointment.

____

____

____

____

____

____

____

____

____

Dental Appointment Records

❑ **DOCTOR VISITS** ❑ **OTHER SERVICES**

Best to use a separate page for each category. Year ____________

Date ____________________ Dr. / Other ____

Purpose ____

____

Treatment Plan ______________ ❑ Pending ❑ Type ________________________________

Treatment Summary ____

❑ Lab ❑ X-ray ❑ Dental Impressions Type _____________________________________

Next Appointment Date ______________________________ Time ______________________

❑ Request copy of Dr.'s report sent to Home and ❑ Other ________________________________

❑ Special Referral Dr. / Other ____

Phone (______) ____ ❑ Referral Slip ❑ X-ray Copy

Purpose ____

____

Visit Summary ____

____

____

____

QUESTIONS - CONCERNS
It is always helpful to have your list ready before your appointment.

____

____

____

____

____

____

____

____

____

Dental Appointment Records

❑ **DOCTOR VISITS** ❑ **OTHER SERVICES**

Best to use a separate page for each category. Year ____________

Date ____________________ Dr. / Other ____

Purpose ____

____

Treatment Plan ______________ ❑ Pending ❑ Type ______________________________

Treatment Summary ____

❑ Lab ❑ X-ray ❑ Dental Impressions Type ______________________________________

Next Appointment Date ______________________________ Time ______________

❑ Request copy of Dr.'s report sent to Home and ❑ Other _______________________

❑ Special Referral Dr. / Other ____

Phone (   ) ____________________________________ ❑ Referral Slip ❑ X-ray Copy

Purpose ____

____

Visit Summary ____

____

____

____

QUESTIONS - CONCERNS
It is always helpful to have your list ready before your appointment.

____

____

____

____

____

____

____

____

____

Dental Appointment Records

❑ **DOCTOR VISITS** ❑ **OTHER SERVICES**

Best to use a separate page for each category. Year ______________

Date ____________________ Dr. / Other ____

Purpose ____

____

Treatment Plan _______________ ❑ Pending ❑ Type _____________________________

Treatment Summary ____

❑ Lab ❑ X-ray ❑ Dental Impressions Type ___________________________________

Next Appointment Date ______________________________ Time ___________________

❑ Request copy of Dr.'s report sent to Home and ❑ Other ____________________________

❑ Special Referral Dr. / Other ____

Phone (______) ______________________________________ ❑ Referral Slip ❑ X-ray Copy

Purpose ____

____

Visit Summary ____

____

____

____

QUESTIONS - CONCERNS
It is always helpful to have your list ready before your appointment.

____

____

____

____

____

____

____

____

____

Dental Appointment Records

❑ **DOCTOR VISITS** ❑ **OTHER SERVICES**

Best to use a separate page for each category. Year ____________

Date ____________________ Dr. / Other ____

Purpose ____

____

Treatment Plan ______________ ❑ Pending ❑ Type _______________________________

Treatment Summary ____

❑ Lab ❑ X-ray ❑ Dental Impressions Type ____

Next Appointment Date ______________________________ Time ______________________

❑ Request copy of Dr.'s report sent to Home and ❑ Other ______________________________

❑ Special Referral Dr. / Other ____

Phone (   ) _______________________________ ❑ Referral Slip ❑ X-ray Copy

Purpose ____

____

Visit Summary ____

____

____

____

QUESTIONS - CONCERNS

It is always helpful to have your list ready before your appointment.

____

____

____

____

____

____

____

____

____

Dental Appointment Records

❑ **DOCTOR VISITS** ❑ **OTHER SERVICES**

Best to use a separate page for each category. Year ____________

Date ____________________ Dr. / Other ____

Purpose ____

____

Treatment Plan ______________ ❑ Pending ❑ Type ______________________________

Treatment Summary ____

❑ Lab ❑ X-ray ❑ Dental Impressions Type ________________________________

Next Appointment Date ______________________________ Time ____________________

❑ Request copy of Dr.'s report sent to Home and ❑ Other ____________________________

❑ Special Referral Dr. / Other ____

Phone (______) _____________________________________ ❑ Referral Slip ❑ X-ray Copy

Purpose ____

____

Visit Summary ____

____

____

____

QUESTIONS - CONCERNS
It is always helpful to have your list ready before your appointment.

____

____

____

____

____

____

____

____

____

Dental Appointment Records

❑ **DOCTOR VISITS** ❑ **OTHER SERVICES**

Best to use a separate page for each category. Year ____________

Date ____________________ Dr. / Other ____

Purpose ____

____

Treatment Plan ______________ ❑ Pending ❑ Type ________________________________

Treatment Summary ____

❑ Lab ❑ X-ray ❑ Dental Impressions Type ____

Next Appointment Date ______________________________ Time ______________________

❑ Request copy of Dr.'s report sent to Home and ❑ Other _________________________________

❑ Special Referral Dr. / Other ____

Phone (   ) _____________________________________ ❑ Referral Slip ❑ X-ray Copy

Purpose ____

____

Visit Summary ____

____

____

____

QUESTIONS - CONCERNS
It is always helpful to have your list ready before your appointment.

____

____

____

____

____

____

____

____

____

Dental Appointment Records

❑ **DOCTOR VISITS** ❑ **OTHER SERVICES**

Best to use a separate page for each category. Year ____________

Date ____________________ Dr. / Other ____

Purpose ____

____

Treatment Plan ______________ ❑ Pending ❑ Type __________________________________

Treatment Summary ____

❑ Lab ❑ X-ray ❑ Dental Impressions Type ______________________________________

Next Appointment Date ______________________________ Time ____________________

❑ Request copy of Dr.'s report sent to Home and ❑ Other ___________________________

❑ Special Referral Dr. / Other ____

Phone (______) ____ ❑ Referral Slip ❑ X-ray Copy

Purpose ____

____

Visit Summary ____

____

____

____

QUESTIONS - CONCERNS

It is always helpful to have your list ready before your appointment.

____

____

____

____

____

____

____

____

____

Dental Appointment Records

❑ **DOCTOR VISITS** ❑ **OTHER SERVICES**

Best to use a separate page for each category. Year ____________

Date ____________________ Dr. / Other ____

Purpose ____

____

Treatment Plan ______________ ❑ Pending ❑ Type ___________________________

Treatment Summary ____

❑ Lab ❑ X-ray ❑ Dental Impressions Type _______________________________________

Next Appointment Date ______________________________ Time ____________________

❑ Request copy of Dr.'s report sent to Home and ❑ Other ___________________________

❑ Special Referral Dr. / Other ____

Phone (______) ______________________________________ ❑ Referral Slip ❑ X-ray Copy

Purpose ____

____

Visit Summary ____

____

____

____

QUESTIONS - CONCERNS
It is always helpful to have your list ready before your appointment.

____

____

____

____

____

____

____

____

____

Dental Appointment Records

❑ **DOCTOR VISITS** ❑ **OTHER SERVICES**

Best to use a separate page for each category. Year ____________

Date ____________________ Dr. / Other ____

Purpose ____

____

Treatment Plan ______________ ❑ Pending ❑ Type ___________________________________

Treatment Summary ____

❑ Lab ❑ X-ray ❑ Dental Impressions Type ____________________________________

Next Appointment Date ______________________________ Time ____________________

❑ Request copy of Dr.'s report sent to Home and ❑ Other ________________________

❑ Special Referral Dr. / Other ____

Phone (   ) ____ ❑ Referral Slip ❑ X-ray Copy

Purpose ____

____

Visit Summary ____

____

____

____

QUESTIONS - CONCERNS
It is always helpful to have your list ready before your appointment.

____

____

____

____

____

____

____

____

____

Dental Appointment Records

❑ **DOCTOR VISITS** ❑ **OTHER SERVICES**

Best to use a separate page for each category. Year ____________

Date ____________________ Dr. / Other ____

Purpose ____

____

Treatment Plan _______________ ❑ Pending ❑ Type ________________________________

Treatment Summary ____

❑ Lab ❑ X-ray ❑ Dental Impressions Type ____

Next Appointment Date ______________________________ Time ______________________

❑ Request copy of Dr.'s report sent to Home and ❑ Other ______________________________

❑ Special Referral Dr. / Other ____

Phone (   ) ______________________________ ❑ Referral Slip ❑ X-ray Copy

Purpose ____

____

Visit Summary ____

____

____

____

QUESTIONS - CONCERNS
It is always helpful to have your list ready before your appointment.

____

____

____

____

____

____

____

____

____

Dental Appointment Records

❑ **DOCTOR VISITS** ❑ **OTHER SERVICES**

Best to use a separate page for each category. Year ____________

Date ____________________ Dr. / Other ____

Purpose ____

____

Treatment Plan ______________ ❑ Pending ❑ Type ___________________________

Treatment Summary ____

❑ Lab ❑ X-ray ❑ Dental Impressions Type ________________________________

Next Appointment Date ______________________________ Time ______________

❑ Request copy of Dr.'s report sent to Home and ❑ Other ____________________

❑ Special Referral Dr. / Other ____

Phone (   ) ____________________________________ ❑ Referral Slip ❑ X-ray Copy

Purpose ____

____

Visit Summary ____

____

____

____

QUESTIONS - CONCERNS
It is always helpful to have your list ready before your appointment.

____

____

____

____

____

____

____

____

____

Dental Appointment Records

❑ **DOCTOR VISITS** ❑ **OTHER SERVICES**

Best to use a separate page for each category. Year ____________

Date __________________ Dr. / Other ______________________________________

Purpose ____

____

Treatment Plan ______________ ❑ Pending ❑ Type ______________________________

Treatment Summary ____

❑ Lab ❑ X-ray ❑ Dental Impressions Type ______________________________________

Next Appointment Date ____________________________ Time ____________________

❑ Request copy of Dr.'s report sent to Home and ❑ Other ______________________________

❑ Special Referral Dr. / Other ____

Phone (   ) ____________________________________ ❑ Referral Slip ❑ X-ray Copy

Purpose ____

____

Visit Summary ____

____

____

____

QUESTIONS - CONCERNS
It is always helpful to have your list ready before your appointment.

____

____

____

____

____

____

____

____

____

LABORATORY WORK * X-RAY LOG AND RECORDS

Log

Maintain a log for easy recall and review.

Records

State the type of test, the reason for it and the results. For your Personal Health Care binder, you may want to request a copy of the report and, or x-rays, depending on the test. This is useful especially for future reference and to assist any professional when evaluating a medical treatment or condition. If the service provider will not release the report to you, then request that it be sent to your physician so that you can obtain a copy.

Notes

Laboratory Work * X-Ray Log

Place a (✓) in the appropriate category.

DATE	TYPE	X-RAY	BLOOD TEST	PROCEDURE	OTHER	COMMENTS

Laboratory Work * X-Ray Log

Place a (✓) in the appropriate category.

DATE	TYPE	X-RAY	BLOOD TEST	PROCEDURE	OTHER	COMMENTS

Laboratory Work * X-Ray Records

❑ **LABORATORY WORK** ❑ **X-RAY**

Best to use a separate page for each category.

Date ____________________ **Phone** (   ) ____________________

Facility ____

Address ____

City ______________________ State ________ Zip ______________

Requested by Dr. ____

Purpose ____

____

Request copy of: ❑ Report ❑ X-rays ❑ Lab Results ❑ Other ______________

Prepare for test: ❑ No ❑ Yes ____________________

Note ____

____

____

____

Date ____________________ Phone (   ) ____________________

Facility ____

Address ____

City ______________________ State ________ Zip ______________

Requested by Dr. ____

Purpose ____

____

Request copy of: ❑ Report ❑ X-rays ❑ Lab Results ❑ Other ______________

Prepare for test: ❑ No ❑ Yes ____________________

Note ____

____

____

____

Laboratory Work * X-Ray

Laboratory Work * X-Ray Records

❑ **LABORATORY WORK** ❑ **X-RAY**

Best to use a separate page for each category.

Date ____________________ **Phone** (   ) ____________________

Facility ____________________

Address ____________________

City ____________________ State ________ Zip ____________________

Requested by Dr. ____________________

Purpose ____________________

____

Request copy of: ❑ Report ❑ X-rays ❑ Lab Results ❑ Other ____________________

Prepare for test: ❑ No ❑ Yes ____________________

Note ____________________

____

____

____

Date ____________________ Phone (   ) ____________________

Facility ____________________

Address ____________________

City ____________________ State ________ Zip ____________________

Requested by Dr. ____________________

Purpose ____________________

____

Request copy of: ❑ Report ❑ X-rays ❑ Lab Results ❑ Other ____________________

Prepare for test: ❑ No ❑ Yes ____________________

Note ____________________

____

____

____

Laboratory Work * X-Ray Records

❑ **LABORATORY WORK** ❑ **X-RAY**

Best to use a separate page for each category.

Date ______________ **Phone** (   ) ______________

Facility ______________

Address ______________

City ______________ State ______ Zip ______________

Requested by Dr. ______________

Purpose ______________

____

Request copy of: ❑ Report ❑ X-rays ❑ Lab Results ❑ Other ______________

Prepare for test: ❑ No ❑ Yes ______________

Note ______________

____

____

____

Date ______________ Phone (   ) ______________

Facility ______________

Address ______________

City ______________ State ______ Zip ______________

Requested by Dr. ______________

Purpose ______________

____

Request copy of: ❑ Report ❑ X-rays ❑ Lab Results ❑ Other ______________

Prepare for test: ❑ No ❑ Yes ______________

Note ______________

____

____

____

Laboratory Work * X-Ray Records

❑ **LABORATORY WORK** ❑ **X-RAY**

Best to use a separate page for each category.

Date ______________ Phone (   ) ______________

Facility ______________

Address ______________

City ______________ State ______ Zip ______

Requested by Dr. ______________

Purpose ______________

____

Request copy of: ❑ Report ❑ X-rays ❑ Lab Results ❑ Other ______________

Prepare for test: ❑ No ❑ Yes ______________

Note ______________

____

____

____

Date ______________ Phone (   ) ______________

Facility ______________

Address ______________

City ______________ State ______ Zip ______

Requested by Dr. ______________

Purpose ______________

____

Request copy of: ❑ Report ❑ X-rays ❑ Lab Results ❑ Other ______________

Prepare for test: ❑ No ❑ Yes ______________

Note ______________

____

____

____

Laboratory Work * X-Ray Records

❑ **LABORATORY WORK** ❑ **X-RAY**

Best to use a separate page for each category.

Date ____________ Phone ( ) ____________

Facility ____________

Address ____________

City ____________ State ______ Zip ____________

Requested by Dr. ____________

Purpose ____________

____

Request copy of: ❑ Report ❑ X-rays ❑ Lab Results ❑ Other ____________

Prepare for test: ❑ No ❑ Yes ____________

Note ____________

____

____

____

Date ____________ Phone ( ) ____________

Facility ____________

Address ____________

City ____________ State ______ Zip ____________

Requested by Dr. ____________

Purpose ____________

____

Request copy of: ❑ Report ❑ X-rays ❑ Lab Results ❑ Other ____________

Prepare for test: ❑ No ❑ Yes ____________

Note ____________

____

____

____

Laboratory Work * X-Ray Records

❑ **LABORATORY WORK** ❑ **X-RAY**

Best to use a separate page for each category.

Date ______________ Phone ( ) ______________________

Facility ____

Address ____

City ______________________ State ______ Zip __________

Requested by Dr. ______________________________________

Purpose ____

____

Request copy of: ❑ Report ❑ X-rays ❑ Lab Results ❑ Other ____________

Prepare for test: ❑ No ❑ Yes _____________________________

Note ____

____

____

____

Date ______________ Phone ( ) ______________________

Facility ____

Address ____

City ______________________ State ______ Zip __________

Requested by Dr. ______________________________________

Purpose ____

____

Request copy of: ❑ Report ❑ X-rays ❑ Lab Results ❑ Other ____________

Prepare for test: ❑ No ❑ Yes _____________________________

Note ____

____

____

____

Laboratory Work * X-Ray Records

❑ **LABORATORY WORK** ❑ **X-RAY**

Best to use a separate page for each category.

Date ____________________ Phone ( ) ______________________________

Facility ____

Address ____

City ______________________________ State ________ Zip ______________

Requested by Dr. ______________________________________

Purpose ____

____

Request copy of: ❑ Report ❑ X-rays ❑ Lab Results ❑ Other ______________

Prepare for test: ❑ No ❑ Yes ______________________________

Note ____

____

____

____

Date ____________________ Phone ( ) ______________________________

Facility ____

Address ____

City ______________________________ State ________ Zip ______________

Requested by Dr. ______________________________________

Purpose ____

____

Request copy of: ❑ Report ❑ X-rays ❑ Lab Results ❑ Other ______________

Prepare for test: ❑ No ❑ Yes ______________________________

Note ____

____

____

____

Laboratory Work * X-Ray Records

❑ **LABORATORY WORK** ❑ **X-RAY**

Best to use a separate page for each category.

Date ____________ Phone (   ) ____________

Facility ____________

Address ____________

City ____________ State ______ Zip ______

Requested by Dr. ____________

Purpose ____________

____

Request copy of: ❑ Report ❑ X-rays ❑ Lab Results ❑ Other ____________

Prepare for test: ❑ No ❑ Yes ____________

Note ____________

____

____

____

Date ____________ Phone (   ) ____________

Facility ____________

Address ____________

City ____________ State ______ Zip ______

Requested by Dr. ____________

Purpose ____________

____

Request copy of: ❑ Report ❑ X-rays ❑ Lab Results ❑ Other ____________

Prepare for test: ❑ No ❑ Yes ____________

Note ____________

____

____

____

Laboratory Work * X-Ray

Laboratory Work * X-Ray Records

❑ **LABORATORY WORK** ❑ **X-RAY**

Best to use a separate page for each category.

Date ____________ **Phone** (____) ____________

Facility ____________

Address ____________

City ____________ State ______ Zip ______

Requested by Dr. ____________

Purpose ____________

____

Request copy of: ❑ Report ❑ X-rays ❑ Lab Results ❑ Other ____________

Prepare for test: ❑ No ❑ Yes ____________

Note ____________

____

____

____

Date ____________ Phone (____) ____________

Facility ____________

Address ____________

City ____________ State ______ Zip ______

Requested by Dr. ____________

Purpose ____________

____

Request copy of: ❑ Report ❑ X-rays ❑ Lab Results ❑ Other ____________

Prepare for test: ❑ No ❑ Yes ____________

Note ____________

____

____

____

Laboratory Work * X-Ray Records

❑ **LABORATORY WORK** ❑ **X-RAY**

Best to use a separate page for each category.

Date ______________ **Phone** (   ) ______________

Facility ______________

Address ______________

City ______________ State ______ Zip ______

Requested by Dr. ______________

Purpose ______________

____

Request copy of: ❑ Report ❑ X-rays ❑ Lab Results ❑ Other ______________

Prepare for test: ❑ No ❑ Yes ______________

Note ______________

____

____

____

Date ______________ Phone (   ) ______________

Facility ______________

Address ______________

City ______________ State ______ Zip ______

Requested by Dr. ______________

Purpose ______________

____

Request copy of: ❑ Report ❑ X-rays ❑ Lab Results ❑ Other ______________

Prepare for test: ❑ No ❑ Yes ______________

Note ______________

____

____

____

Laboratory Work * X-Ray Records

❑ **LABORATORY WORK** ❑ **X-RAY**

Best to use a separate page for each category.

Date ______________ Phone (   ) ______________

Facility ______________

Address ______________

City ______________ State ______ Zip ______________

Requested by Dr. ______________

Purpose ______________

____

Request copy of: ❑ Report ❑ X-rays ❑ Lab Results ❑ Other ______________

Prepare for test: ❑ No ❑ Yes ______________

Note ______________

____

____

____

Date ______________ Phone (   ) ______________

Facility ______________

Address ______________

City ______________ State ______ Zip ______________

Requested by Dr. ______________

Purpose ______________

____

Request copy of: ❑ Report ❑ X-rays ❑ Lab Results ❑ Other ______________

Prepare for test: ❑ No ❑ Yes ______________

Note ______________

____

____

____

Laboratory Work * X-Ray

Laboratory Work * X-Ray Records

❑ **LABORATORY WORK** ❑ **X-RAY**

Best to use a separate page for each category.

Date ______________________ Phone (   ) ______________________

Facility ______________________

Address ______________________

City ______________________ State ________ Zip ______________

Requested by Dr. ______________________

Purpose ______________________

____

Request copy of: ❑ Report ❑ X-rays ❑ Lab Results ❑ Other ______________

Prepare for test: ❑ No ❑ Yes ______________________

Note ______________________

____

____

____

Date ______________________ Phone (   ) ______________________

Facility ______________________

Address ______________________

City ______________________ State ________ Zip ______________

Requested by Dr. ______________________

Purpose ______________________

____

Request copy of: ❑ Report ❑ X-rays ❑ Lab Results ❑ Other ______________

Prepare for test: ❑ No ❑ Yes ______________________

Note ______________________

____

____

____

Laboratory Work * X-Ray Records

❑ **LABORATORY WORK** ❑ **X-RAY**

Best to use a separate page for each category.

Date ____________________ **Phone** (   ) ____________________

Facility ____________________

Address ____________________

City ____________________ State ________ Zip ____________________

Requested by Dr. ____________________

Purpose ____________________

____

Request copy of: ❑ Report ❑ X-rays ❑ Lab Results ❑ Other ____________________

Prepare for test: ❑ No ❑ Yes ____________________

Note ____________________

____

____

____

Date ____________________ Phone (   ) ____________________

Facility ____________________

Address ____________________

City ____________________ State ________ Zip ____________________

Requested by Dr. ____________________

Purpose ____________________

____

Request copy of: ❑ Report ❑ X-rays ❑ Lab Results ❑ Other ____________________

Prepare for test: ❑ No ❑ Yes ____________________

Note ____________________

____

____

____

Laboratory Work * X-Ray Records

❑ **LABORATORY WORK** ❑ **X-RAY**

Best to use a separate page for each category.

Date ____________ **Phone** ( ) ____________

Facility ____________

Address ____________

City ____________ State ______ Zip ______

Requested by Dr. ____________

Purpose ____________

____

Request copy of: ❑ Report ❑ X-rays ❑ Lab Results ❑ Other ____________

Prepare for test: ❑ No ❑ Yes ____________

Note ____________

____

____

____

Date ____________ Phone ( ) ____________

Facility ____________

Address ____________

City ____________ State ______ Zip ______

Requested by Dr. ____________

Purpose ____________

____

Request copy of: ❑ Report ❑ X-rays ❑ Lab Results ❑ Other ____________

Prepare for test: ❑ No ❑ Yes ____________

Note ____________

____

____

____

Immunizations * Injections Log and Records

Log

Maintain a log for easy recall and review.

Records

These records are needed throughout your lifetime.

There are certain immunizations recommended by your physician for ages 0-6 years, 7-18 years, adult and seniors. Check with your health care providers for what you may need for your age group.

When traveling be sure to find out what immunizations are required.

For more information check with the Health Services Foundation and Center for Disease Control in your country.

Note: Children and adults with special risk factors and, or allergies may require additional or alternative immunizations. Always discuss with your physician the risks involved with any immunizations and treatments.

Notes

Immunization Log

Place the month and year in the box. If you observe a reaction to the immunization complete the *'Immunization Record'* with the pertinent information needed to assist the physician. Also, mark the box with an *'R'* next to the date to know which immunization showed a reaction.

Check with your Physician at any age if you need the following immunizations.

Chickenpox (VZV)

Diphtheria, Tetanus, Pertussis (DTaP/Td)

Haemophilus influenzae type b (Hib)

Hepatitis A (HepA)

Hepatitis B (HepB)

Human Papillomavirus (HPV)

Inactivated Poliovirus (IPV)

Influenza

Measles, Mumps, Rubella (MMR)

Meningococcal (MCV4)

Immunization Log

Place the month and year in the box. If you observe a reaction to the immunization complete the *'Immunization Record'* with the pertinent information needed to assist the physician. Also, mark the box with an *'R'* next to the date to know which immunization showed a reaction.

Check with your Physician at any age if you need the following immunizations.

Pneumococcal (PPV)

Rotavirus (Rota)

Tuberculosis (TB Test)

Varicella

Other: Type ______________________

Other: Type ______________________

Other: Type ______________________

Other: Type ______________________

Other: Type ______________________

Other: Type ______________________

Immunization * Injection Records

Date ____________ Doctor / Clinic ____________

Type ____________

Purpose ____________

Reaction ____________

Counteraction ____________

Instructions ____________

____

____

Date ____________ Doctor / Clinic ____________

Type ____________

Purpose ____________

Reaction ____________

Counteraction ____________

Instructions ____________

____

____

Date ____________ Doctor / Clinic ____________

Type ____________

Purpose ____________

Reaction ____________

Counteraction ____________

Instructions ____________

____

Immunization * Injection Records

Date ______________ Doctor / Clinic ______________

Type ______________

Purpose ______________

Reaction ______________

Counteraction ______________

Instructions ______________

Date ______________ Doctor / Clinic ______________

Type ______________

Purpose ______________

Reaction ______________

Counteraction ______________

Instructions ______________

Date ______________ Doctor / Clinic ______________

Type ______________

Purpose ______________

Reaction ______________

Counteraction ______________

Instructions ______________

Immunization * Injection Records

Date ______________________ Doctor / Clinic ______________________

Type ______________________

Purpose ______________________

Reaction ______________________

Counteraction ______________________

Instructions ______________________

____

____

Date ______________________ Doctor / Clinic ______________________

Type ______________________

Purpose ______________________

Reaction ______________________

Counteraction ______________________

Instructions ______________________

____

____

Date ______________________ Doctor / Clinic ______________________

Type ______________________

Purpose ______________________

Reaction ______________________

Counteraction ______________________

Instructions ______________________

____

Immunization * Injection Records

Date ________________ Doctor / Clinic ________________

Type ________________

Purpose ________________

Reaction ________________

Counteraction ________________

Instructions ________________

____

____

Date ________________ Doctor / Clinic ________________

Type ________________

Purpose ________________

Reaction ________________

Counteraction ________________

Instructions ________________

____

____

Date ________________ Doctor / Clinic ________________

Type ________________

Purpose ________________

Reaction ________________

Counteraction ________________

Instructions ________________

____

Immunization * Injection Records

Date ______________________ Doctor / Clinic ____

Type ____

Purpose ____

Reaction ____

Counteraction ____

Instructions ____

____

____

Date ______________________ Doctor / Clinic ____

Type ____

Purpose ____

Reaction ____

Counteraction ____

Instructions ____

____

____

Date ______________________ Doctor / Clinic ____

Type ____

Purpose ____

Reaction ____

Counteraction ____

Instructions ____

____

Immunization * Injection Records

Date ____________ Doctor / Clinic ____________

Type ____________

Purpose ____________

Reaction ____________

Counteraction ____________

Instructions ____________

____

____

Date ____________ Doctor / Clinic ____________

Type ____________

Purpose ____________

Reaction ____________

Counteraction ____________

Instructions ____________

____

____

Date ____________ Doctor / Clinic ____________

Type ____________

Purpose ____________

Reaction ____________

Counteraction ____________

Instructions ____________

____

Service Agencies

This information is helpful when utilizing services from a particular program, assocation or provider. (i.e., funding sources, physical therapy, nutritionist, transportation, educational programs, etc.)

This section may be utilized at various stages of your life.

Notes

Service Agencies

❑ **SERVICE AGENCIES** ❑ **Other**

Best to use a separate page for each category. Add the address and phone numbers in the address section. Also, collect business cards for easy reference.

Date ____________________

Agency ____________________

Address ____________________

City ____________________ State ______ Zip ____________________

Phone (______) ____________________

Provider ____________________

Purpose ____________________

Preparation ____________________

❑ Fees ____________ ❑ Insurance ____________ ❑ Other ____________

Next Appointment Date ____________ Time ____________

Summary ____________________

____

Date ____________________

Agency ____________________

Address ____________________

City ____________________ State ______ Zip ____________________

Phone (______) ____________________

Provider ____________________

Purpose ____________________

Preparation ____________________

❑ Fees ____________ ❑ Insurance ____________ ❑ Other ____________

Next Appointment Date ____________ Time ____________

Summary ____________________

____

Service Agencies

❑ **SERVICE AGENCIES** ❑ **Other**

Best to use a separate page for each category. Add the address and phone numbers in the address section. Also, collect business cards for easy reference.

Date ______________________________

Agency ______________________________

Address ______________________________

City ______________________ State ______ Zip ______________

Phone (______) ______________________________

Provider ______________________________

Purpose ______________________________

Preparation ______________________________

❑ Fees ____________ ❑ Insurance ______________ ❑ Other ______________

Next Appointment Date ______________ Time ______________

Summary ______________________________

____

Date ______________________________

Agency ______________________________

Address ______________________________

City ______________________ State ______ Zip ______________

Phone (______) ______________________________

Provider ______________________________

Purpose ______________________________

Preparation ______________________________

❑ Fees ____________ ❑ Insurance ______________ ❑ Other ______________

Next Appointment Date ______________ Time ______________

Summary ______________________________

____

Service Agencies

❑ **SERVICE AGENCIES** ❑ **Other**

Best to use a separate page for each category. Add the address and phone numbers in the address section. Also, collect business cards for easy reference.

Date ______________________________

Agency ______________________________

Address ______________________________

City ____________________ State ______ Zip ____________

Phone (______) ______________________________

Provider ______________________________

Purpose ______________________________

Preparation ______________________________

❑ Fees ____________ ❑ Insurance ____________ ❑ Other ____________

Next Appointment Date ____________ Time ____________

Summary ______________________________

____

Date ______________________________

Agency ______________________________

Address ______________________________

City ____________________ State ______ Zip ____________

Phone (______) ______________________________

Provider ______________________________

Purpose ______________________________

Preparation ______________________________

❑ Fees ____________ ❑ Insurance ____________ ❑ Other ____________

Next Appointment Date ____________ Time ____________

Summary ______________________________

____

Service Agencies

❑ **SERVICE AGENCIES** ❑ **Other**

Best to use a separate page for each category. Add the address and phone numbers in the address section. Also, collect business cards for easy reference.

Date ______________________________

Agency ______________________________

Address ______________________________

City ____________________ State ______ Zip ____________

Phone (______) ______________________________

Provider ______________________________

Purpose ______________________________

Preparation ______________________________

❑ Fees ____________ ❑ Insurance ______________ ❑ Other ____________

Next Appointment Date ____________ Time ______________

Summary ______________________________

____

Date ______________________________

Agency ______________________________

Address ______________________________

City ____________________ State ______ Zip ____________

Phone (______) ______________________________

Provider ______________________________

Purpose ______________________________

Preparation ______________________________

❑ Fees ____________ ❑ Insurance ______________ ❑ Other ____________

Next Appointment Date ____________ Time ______________

Summary ______________________________

____

Service Agencies

❑ **SERVICE AGENCIES** ❑ **Other**

Best to use a separate page for each category. Add the address and phone numbers in the address section. Also, collect business cards for easy reference.

Date ______________________________

Agency ______________________________

Address ______________________________

City ______________________ State ______ Zip ______________

Phone (______) ______________________________

Provider ______________________________

Purpose ______________________________

Preparation ______________________________

❑ Fees ____________ ❑ Insurance ______________ ❑ Other ______________

Next Appointment Date ______________ Time ______________________

Summary ______________________________

____

Date ______________________________

Agency ______________________________

Address ______________________________

City ______________________ State ______ Zip ______________

Phone (______) ______________________________

Provider ______________________________

Purpose ______________________________

Preparation ______________________________

❑ Fees ____________ ❑ Insurance ______________ ❑ Other ______________

Next Appointment Date ______________ Time ______________________

Summary ______________________________

____

Service Agencies

❑ **SERVICE AGENCIES** ❑ **Other**

Best to use a separate page for each category. Add the address and phone numbers in the address section. Also, collect business cards for easy reference.

Date ______________________

Agency ______________________

Address ______________________

City ______________ State ______ Zip ______________

Phone (______) ______________________

Provider ______________________

Purpose ______________________

Preparation ______________________

❑ Fees ______________ ❑ Insurance ______________ ❑ Other ______________

Next Appointment Date ______________ Time ______________

Summary ______________________

____

Date ______________________

Agency ______________________

Address ______________________

City ______________ State ______ Zip ______________

Phone (______) ______________________

Provider ______________________

Purpose ______________________

Preparation ______________________

❑ Fees ______________ ❑ Insurance ______________ ❑ Other ______________

Next Appointment Date ______________ Time ______________

Summary ______________________

____

Name & Address Index

Keep the phone numbers and addresses of anyone who is assisting you with your medical and dental health care.

Notes

Name & Address Index

Listing from ______ to ______

❑ DOCTOR ❑ HOSPITAL ❑ SERVICE ❑ AGENCY ❑ THERAPIST

You may want to group by discipline or service per page.

Name ______________________ Phone (______) ______________________
Specialty Field ______________________ Fax (______) ______________________
Nurse ______________________ Other ______________________
Hospital ______________________ E-mail ______________________
Clinic / Dept. ____
Address ______________________ Ste/Room ______________________
City ______________ State __________ Zip ______________________
Note ____

Name ______________________ Phone (______) ______________________
Specialty Field ______________________ Fax (______) ______________________
Nurse ______________________ Other ______________________
Hospital ______________________ E-mail ______________________
Clinic / Dept. ____
Address ______________________ Ste/Room ______________________
City ______________ State __________ Zip ______________________
Note ____

Name ______________________ Phone (______) ______________________
Specialty Field ______________________ Fax (______) ______________________
Nurse ______________________ Other ______________________
Hospital ______________________ E-mail ______________________
Clinic / Dept. ____
Address ______________________ Ste/Room ______________________
City ______________ State __________ Zip ______________________
Note ____

Name ______________________ Phone (______) ______________________
Specialty Field ______________________ Fax (______) ______________________
Nurse ______________________ Other ______________________
Hospital ______________________ E-mail ______________________
Clinic / Dept. ____
Address ______________________ Ste/Room ______________________
City ______________ State __________ Zip ______________________
Note ____

Name & Address Index

Listing from ______ to ______

❑ DOCTOR ❑ HOSPITAL ❑ SERVICE ❑ AGENCY ❑ THERAPIST

You may want to group by discipline or service per page.

Name ______ Phone ( ) ______
Specialty Field ______ Fax ( ) ______
Nurse ______ Other ______
Hospital ______ E-mail ______
Clinic / Dept. ______
Address ______ Ste/Room ______
City ______ State ______ Zip ______
Note ______

Name ______ Phone ( ) ______
Specialty Field ______ Fax ( ) ______
Nurse ______ Other ______
Hospital ______ E-mail ______
Clinic / Dept. ______
Address ______ Ste/Room ______
City ______ State ______ Zip ______
Note ______

Name ______ Phone ( ) ______
Specialty Field ______ Fax ( ) ______
Nurse ______ Other ______
Hospital ______ E-mail ______
Clinic / Dept. ______
Address ______ Ste/Room ______
City ______ State ______ Zip ______
Note ______

Name ______ Phone ( ) ______
Specialty Field ______ Fax ( ) ______
Nurse ______ Other ______
Hospital ______ E-mail ______
Clinic / Dept. ______
Address ______ Ste/Room ______
City ______ State ______ Zip ______
Note ______

Name & Address Index

Listing from ______ to ______

❑ DOCTOR ❑ HOSPITAL ❑ SERVICE ❑ AGENCY ❑ THERAPIST

You may want to group by discipline or service per page.

Name ______________________ Phone ( ) ______________________
Specialty Field ______________________ Fax ( ) ______________________
Nurse ______________________ Other ______________________
Hospital ______________________ E-mail ______________________
Clinic / Dept. ______________________
Address ______________________ Ste/Room ______________________
City ____________ State ____________ Zip ______________________
Note ______________________

Name ______________________ Phone ( ) ______________________
Specialty Field ______________________ Fax ( ) ______________________
Nurse ______________________ Other ______________________
Hospital ______________________ E-mail ______________________
Clinic / Dept. ______________________
Address ______________________ Ste/Room ______________________
City ____________ State ____________ Zip ______________________
Note ______________________

Name ______________________ Phone ( ) ______________________
Specialty Field ______________________ Fax ( ) ______________________
Nurse ______________________ Other ______________________
Hospital ______________________ E-mail ______________________
Clinic / Dept. ______________________
Address ______________________ Ste/Room ______________________
City ____________ State ____________ Zip ______________________
Note ______________________

Name ______________________ Phone ( ) ______________________
Specialty Field ______________________ Fax ( ) ______________________
Nurse ______________________ Other ______________________
Hospital ______________________ E-mail ______________________
Clinic / Dept. ______________________
Address ______________________ Ste/Room ______________________
City ____________ State ____________ Zip ______________________
Note ______________________

Name & Address Index

Listing from ______ to ______

❑ **DOCTOR** ❑ **HOSPITAL** ❑ **SERVICE** ❑ **AGENCY** ❑ **THERAPIST**

You may want to group by discipline or service per page.

Name ______ Phone ( ) ______
Specialty Field ______ Fax ( ) ______
Nurse ______ Other ______
Hospital ______ E-mail ______
Clinic / Dept. ______
Address ______ Ste/Room ______
City ______ State ______ Zip ______
Note ______

Name ______ Phone ( ) ______
Specialty Field ______ Fax ( ) ______
Nurse ______ Other ______
Hospital ______ E-mail ______
Clinic / Dept. ______
Address ______ Ste/Room ______
City ______ State ______ Zip ______
Note ______

Name ______ Phone ( ) ______
Specialty Field ______ Fax ( ) ______
Nurse ______ Other ______
Hospital ______ E-mail ______
Clinic / Dept. ______
Address ______ Ste/Room ______
City ______ State ______ Zip ______
Note ______

Name ______ Phone ( ) ______
Specialty Field ______ Fax ( ) ______
Nurse ______ Other ______
Hospital ______ E-mail ______
Clinic / Dept. ______
Address ______ Ste/Room ______
City ______ State ______ Zip ______
Note ______

Name & Address Index

Listing from ______ to ______

❑ DOCTOR ❑ HOSPITAL ❑ SERVICE ❑ AGENCY ❑ THERAPIST

You may want to group by discipline or service per page.

Name ______ Phone ( )
Specialty Field ______ Fax ( )
Nurse ______ Other ______
Hospital ______ E-mail ______
Clinic / Dept. ______
Address ______ Ste/Room ______
City ______ State ______ Zip ______
Note ______

Name ______ Phone ( )
Specialty Field ______ Fax ( )
Nurse ______ Other ______
Hospital ______ E-mail ______
Clinic / Dept. ______
Address ______ Ste/Room ______
City ______ State ______ Zip ______
Note ______

Name ______ Phone ( )
Specialty Field ______ Fax ( )
Nurse ______ Other ______
Hospital ______ E-mail ______
Clinic / Dept. ______
Address ______ Ste/Room ______
City ______ State ______ Zip ______
Note ______

Name ______ Phone ( )
Specialty Field ______ Fax ( )
Nurse ______ Other ______
Hospital ______ E-mail ______
Clinic / Dept. ______
Address ______ Ste/Room ______
City ______ State ______ Zip ______
Note ______

Name & Address Index

Listing from ______ to ______

❑ **DOCTOR** ❑ **HOSPITAL** ❑ **SERVICE** ❑ **AGENCY** ❑ **THERAPIST**

You may want to group by discipline or service per page.

Name ____________________ Phone (______) ____________

Specialty Field ____________________ Fax (______) ____________

Nurse ____________________ Other ____________

Hospital ____________________ E-mail ____________

Clinic / Dept. ____________________

Address ____________________ Ste/Room ____________

City ____________ State ________ Zip ____________

Note ____________________

Name ____________________ Phone (______) ____________

Specialty Field ____________________ Fax (______) ____________

Nurse ____________________ Other ____________

Hospital ____________________ E-mail ____________

Clinic / Dept. ____________________

Address ____________________ Ste/Room ____________

City ____________ State ________ Zip ____________

Note ____________________

Name ____________________ Phone (______) ____________

Specialty Field ____________________ Fax (______) ____________

Nurse ____________________ Other ____________

Hospital ____________________ E-mail ____________

Clinic / Dept. ____________________

Address ____________________ Ste/Room ____________

City ____________ State ________ Zip ____________

Note ____________________

Name ____________________ Phone (______) ____________

Specialty Field ____________________ Fax (______) ____________

Nurse ____________________ Other ____________

Hospital ____________________ E-mail ____________

Clinic / Dept. ____________________

Address ____________________ Ste/Room ____________

City ____________ State ________ Zip ____________

Note ____________________

RESOURCES

This section contains a request for information, an endorsement sheet and an emergency card, all for your convenience.

Notes

Cut

Complete your information, cut along dotted line.

INFORMATION REQUEST

To order additional copies, current pricing, or for more information please return this page to the address listed below or go to the web site at www.LCPBooks.com.

Name ______________________________

Company ______________________________

Address ______________________ Apt/Ste. ______________________

City ______________ State ______ Zip ______ Country ______________

Phone (   ) ______________________ Cell (   ) ______________________

Fax (   ) ______________________________

E-mail ______________________________

I am interested in the following:

- ❑ Personal Medical Journal
- ❑ My Personal Medical Journal
- ❑ Allergy Card
- ❑ Cover ~ ❑ ___Blue ❑ ___Black ❑ ___Burgundy
- ❑ Emergency Medical Card
- ❑ Medical History Summary
- ❑ Bulk Rate
- ❑ Bulk Purchase

ꝏ

❑ I am arranging a meeting and would like to invite Gloria Lopez to be a speaker.

Event ______________________________

Topic ______________________________

Date ______________________ Time ______________________

ꝏ

If you have any comments please feel free to add them here and return this form.

____

____

____

ꝏ

We would appreciate your endorsement of the jounal, please complete and return the following page.

Mail to: **Life Cycles Publishing, Inc.**
2937 Veneman Ave., Ste. A105
Modesto, CA 95356

Online: **www.LCPBooks.com**
Phone: (888) 338.0103
Fax: (209) 338.0103

Cut

Resources

Endorsement Sheet

Please keep brief preferably 1-3 lines.

____

____

____

____

How would you like your name to appear?

Name ______________________________

Title ______________________________

Business ______________________________

Other ______________________________

I give permission to use the above statement in:

- ❑ All literature, to include the following:
  - ❑ Book either on the front or the back cover, possibly within the text content.
  - ❑ Web - Internet
  - ❑ Media
  - ❑ Newspapers, Magazines, Periodicals
  - ❑ I would like to be kept informed when my name will be applied to anything.
  - ❑ I want to limit this endorsement to the following:

Signed ______________________ Date ______________________

Please either:

1. Mail to: Life Cycles Publishing
   2937 Veneman Ave., Ste. A105
   Modesto, CA 95356

2. Fax to: (209) 338.0103

Should you have any questions, please do not hesitate to contact me at (209) 577.4200 or (888) 338.0103.

Thank You.

Gloria A. Lopez
CEO/Author

Resources

Cut

Complete your information, cut along dotted line.

Cut

Complete your information, cut along dotted lines, fold and place into your wallet.

Personal Emergency Card

Name ______________________________

Address ______________ Apt. __________

City/State/Zip ______________ Country ______

Phone (   ) ____________ Fax (   ) ________

Email ______________________________

Physician ______________________________

Dr. Phone # (   ) ______________________

Emergency Contact ____________ State ____ Zip ______

Phone # (   ) ______________________

Life Cycles Publishing Inc. www.LCPBooks.com (888) 338.0103

Medications

	Type	Dose	Frequency
1.			
2.			
3.			
4.			
5.			
6.			
7.			

Life Cycles Publishing Inc. www.LCPBooks.com (888) 338.0103

Personal Emergency Card

Name ______________________________

Address ______________ Apt. __________

City/State/Zip ______________ Country ______

Phone (   ) ____________ Fax (   ) ________

Email ______________________________

Physician ______________________________

Dr. Phone # (   ) ______________________

Emergency Contact ____________ State ____ Zip ______

Phone # (   ) ______________________

Life Cycles Publishing Inc. www.LCPBooks.com (888) 338.0103

Medications

Type Dose Frequency

1. 2. 3. 4. 5. 6. 7.

Life Cycles Publishing Inc. www.LCPBooks.com (888) 338.0103

Cut fold Cut Cut fold Cut Cut Cut Cut

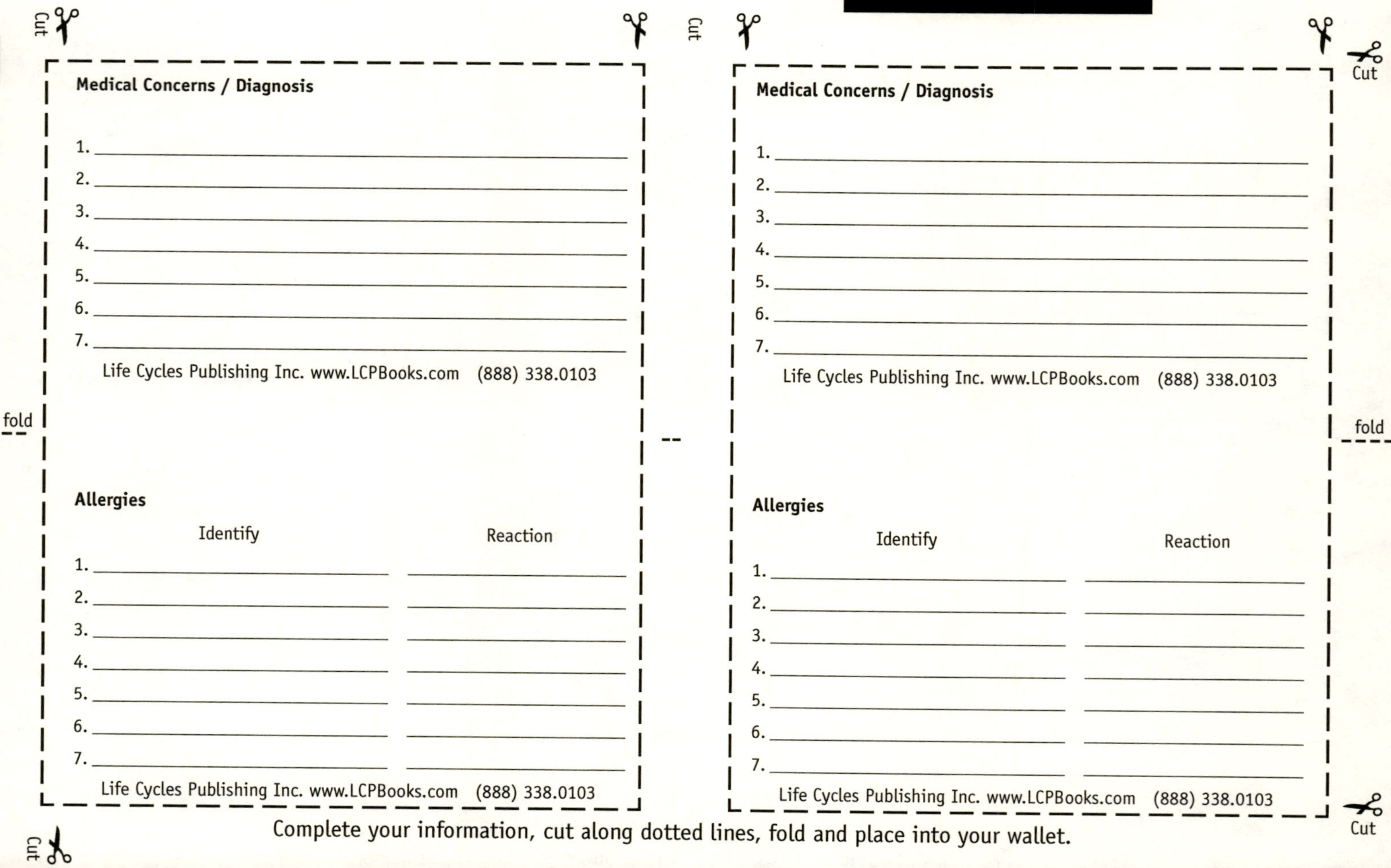

Cut

Cut

Medical Concerns / Diagnosis

1. ______
2. ______
3. ______
4. ______
5. ______
6. ______
7. ______

Life Cycles Publishing Inc. www.LCPBooks.com (888) 338.0103

fold

Allergies

	Identify	Reaction
1.		
2.		
3.		
4.		
5.		
6.		
7.		

Life Cycles Publishing Inc. www.LCPBooks.com (888) 338.0103

Medical Concerns / Diagnosis

1. ______
2. ______
3. ______
4. ______
5. ______
6. ______
7. ______

Life Cycles Publishing Inc. www.LCPBooks.com (888) 338.0103

fold

Allergies

	Identify	Reaction
1.		
2.		
3.		
4.		
5.		
6.		
7.		

Life Cycles Publishing Inc. www.LCPBooks.com (888) 338.0103

Cut

Cut

Cut

Complete your information, cut along dotted lines, fold and place into your wallet.

The Author

For over 35 years, Gloria A. Lopez has worked with families whose children have disabilities, and also, with adults diagnosed with medical conditions later in life. The Personal Medical Journal grew out of her life experiences. It is now designed to help you, or your caregiver, take control of your medical needs.

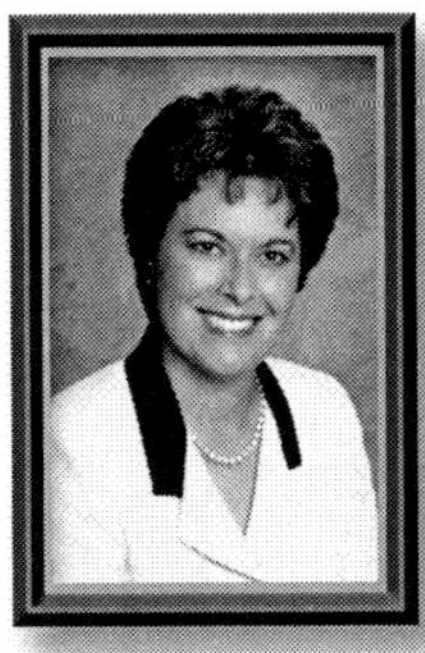

Her son Michael, was born with Spina Bifida, a neural tube birth defect. He was the inspiration that created the first version of the Personal Medical Journal. It continues to help her keep track of Michael's comprehensive medical information, eliminating the need for memorizing and reiterating his medical history. She also used the journal for her two daughters, who although healthy, now have a concise, easily accessible Personal Medical Journals of their own. Additionally, it provides medical professionals easy and accurate access to pertinent information in case of an emergency.

Gloria has helped develop several support groups for parents and the local community, including a group for parents experiencing the trauma of having a newborn in a neonatal hospital unit. She has assisted in developing a program to mainstream children with disabilities into local school districts of Santa Clara County, California.

As a speaker, a medical conference planner, an advocate for child and parental rights, and a program developer on a community, state and national level, Gloria has been active with many issues affecting the disabled. She was a founder and Administrative Director of the Spina Bifida Association of California and continues to work with medical professionals on disability awareness and program development.

Gloria has shown countless families and individuals how to put together their own Personal Medical Journals. It has assisted them in maintaining accurate records and has encouraged them to take an active role in their medical care.

ꝏ

Gloria Ann Lopez

Notes

Notes

Notes

My Personal Medical Journal

- User friendly with sectioned categories that help you keep track of all doctors comments, instructions, medications, etc.
- Helps you to fill out the medical forms when visiting a new physician or medical facility.
- It is a must to take with you when traveling.
- In case of an emergency and you are unable to speak for yourself, your information is documented and at your finger tips.
- It also has information to help you form a list of questions to ask your doctor at the time of your appointment.

Every one of your medical professionals have a piece of your medical history.
It is important that you always have access to your complete health care records.
YOU are the single source for all your health and medical information.

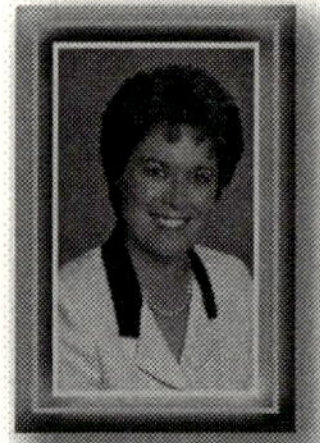

My Personal Medical Journal guides you in maintaining your medical records and participating with your health care professionals.

Gloria Lopez

"It's imperative for the Dentist as well as the Physician to know his/her patient's medical condition as exact and complete as possible. With the help of such concise information medical disasters can be averted and proper treatment be rendered".

Lawrence J. Sarkis, D.D.S., Ripon, CA

Ms. Cordle Hits the Mark

This Journal manages to cover all of the subjects you may need to refer to when you are traveling. It is very detailed and may seem a bit over whelming to record all of the information at first so I would recommend starting with your most current information and work back. It is amazing how many memories come back when you flip through the journal as well as information that you need to acquire. Each member of the family should have their own and it should be the first item packed for a trip. If you carry any kind of an organizer this journal should be kept with it. In case of an emergency the information that is kept in the journal could save a lot of time.

S.Q. Lund, CA

LIFECYCLES
PUBLISHING, INC
1.888.338.0103
WWW.LCPBOOKS.COM